OXFORD MEDICAL

# CHILDHOOD LEUKAEMIA

## the**facts**

### Second Edition

# the**facts**
## ALSO AVAILABLE IN THE SERIES

# CHILDHOOD LEUKAEMIA

## the**facts**

**John S. Lilleyman**

Professor of Paediatric Oncology,
*St Bartholomew's and the Royal London School of*
*Medicine and Dentistry, The Royal London Hospital,*
*Whitechapel, London, UK*

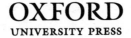

**OXFORD**
UNIVERSITY PRESS

# OXFORD

UNIVERSITY PRESS

Great Clarendon Street, Oxford OX2 6DP

Oxford University Press is a department of the University of Oxford.
It furthers the University's objective of excellence in research, scholarship,
and education by publishing worldwide in

Oxford New York

Athens Auckland Bangkok Bogotá Buenos Aires Calcutta
Cape Town Chennai Dar es Salaam Delhi Florence Hong Kong Istanbul
Karachi Kuala Lumpur Madrid Melbourne Mexico City Mumbai
Nairobi Paris São Paulo Singapore Taipei Tokyo Toronto Warsaw

and associated companies in Berlin Ibadan

Oxford is a registered trade mark of Oxford University Press
in the UK and in certain other countries

Published in the United States
by Oxford University Press Inc., New York

First edition published 1994
Second edition published 2000

A catalogue record for this book is available from the British Library

Library of Congress Cataloging in Publication Data
Lilleyman, J. S.
Chilhood leukaemia/John S. Lilleyman.
(The facts)
Includes bibliographical references.
ISBN 0 19 263142 X

1. Leukemia in children Popular works. I. Title. II. Series: Facts (Oxford, England)

RJ416.L4L549    2000     618.92'99419–dc21      99–39047

Typeset by EXPO Holdings, Malaysia

Printed in Great Britain
on acid-free paper by
Biddles Ltd, Guildford & King's Lynn

# Preface to the second edition

Exactly 5 years have passed since the first edition of this book was written. During that time several parallel tracks of scientific and medical progress have influenced our understanding of the way the various leukaemias develop, what might be involved in the cause of some types, and how better to treat them. We also have new tools to combat the complications of ever more intensive chemotherapy programmes, and the ground rules of bone marrow transplantation have moved.

Despite this progress, of every 10 children who develop leukaemia three or four will still die of the disease even if they are given the most up to date treatment in the best-equipped hospitals in the world. Different types of leukaemia have different outlooks, of course, but there is no room for complacency and careful clinical trials to improve treatment are as important as ever. Also, growing attention is being focused on the increasing number of long survivors. Will their leukaemia return after many years? Are they at increased risk of other cancers? Will they have children? Will their children get leukaemia?

This new edition attempts to explain the new science, the new treatment strategies, and the new worries for parents and the children themselves. The book has been restructured into 16 smaller chapters, some of which are completely new and all of which have been overhauled and updated. Important new words like 'oncogene' and 'apoptosis' appear. Also new to this edition is the concept of 'shared care' between children's cancer units and local district hospitals.

There is expanded discussion and explanation of the need for randomized trials and other experimental treatments being explored in leukaemia, together with the ethical dilemmas and the problems of informed consent that they raise. Finally there is more detailed consideration of the late effects of otherwise successful treatment.

Some things do not change. The Damocles syndrome is as real as ever. The difficulty in coping and getting on with everyday life during and after the experience of leukaemia in a child remains just as great, whether treatment is successful or not. And factual information to help alleviate fear of the unknown will always be needed. So here, again, is an attempt partially to fill that need. But remember, every child with leukaemia is unique and this book only aims to provide broad background knowledge. It cannot supplant the personal advice from a child's physician.

J. S. L.

*London*
2000

# Preface to the first edition

Leukaemia is one of the most frightening words in the English language. Everyone has heard of it. Everyone knows it is a potentially fatal disease. Every now and then there is a major news item about a clue to its cause being found in the environment or of a 'breakthrough' in treatment. These fragments of often distorted information sink into the subconscious ready to surface when the unthinkable happens and the topic takes on a personal urgency.

In fact leukaemia is not a single disease, but rather a group of several disorders that produce broadly similar symptoms. Some are very similar and closely related, others are quite different. Though rare, collectively they form the commonest life-threatening disorder in childhood. Their complexity is still being unravelled as new techniques for the laboratory study of blood and bone marrow are developed, and steady progress in treatment has also been made over the last 45 years. Children with the most responsive types of leukaemia now stand an 80–90 per cent chance of being cured. Others are much less fortunate, but there are no longer any sufferers for whom long-term survival rates are zero.

Once the initial shock of being told the diagnosis starts to recede, questions flood into parents' minds, some rational, some not. What causes it? Is it our fault? Is it inherited? Can our other children catch it? There may be some anger, either directed towards delays in the disease being discovered ('no one would listen, I *said* there was something wrong') or undirected ('it all seems so *unfair*'). Despair is common ('we must have the best treatment whatever it costs'), as is guilt ('I feel we must be responsible in some way'). These reactions and the later struggle to understand the intricate treatment programmes and their complications require a continual supply of factual information and moral support from the team of doctors, nurses, and others working in the leukaemia centre.

The advice given to families by such teams is, of course, irreplaceable as it relates to a particular individual and is focused in a way that general information available from other sources could never be. But there is also a valuable place for informed books and articles about childhood leukaemia for non-specialists. Such publications are helpful as background reading both for relatives of children with the disease and those involved with them such as nurses, general practice teams, teachers, social workers, health visitors, and community workers.

## Preface to the first edition

Continuing in the established and popular format of the Oxford University Press 'Facts' series, what follows is a short but, I hope, comprehensive book designed to explain in simple terms what childhood leukaemia is, who gets it, how it manifests itself, what the various types have in common, and how they differ. Also described are the current programmes of treatment, how they have evolved, the complications that can arise, both in the early days and later after treatment has finished, and the psychological and social impact of the ordeal on parents and children. The place of bone marrow transplantation is discussed and future directions for research into understanding both the nature of the disorder and its management are briefly considered. There is a preliminary section with some background scientific detail about cells, cancer, the blood, and bone marrow. This may take a little effort to get through, but has been included because it helps to make sense of how the different leukaemias behave and how they respond to treatment, and also because it provides the answers to many of the questions repeatedly asked about why this or that happens or what it means when the blood count is 'low'.

In other words, the contents are influenced by the many conversations I have had over the years with leukaemia sufferers, their parents, brothers, sisters, grandparents, uncles, aunts, and friends. All have taught me a great deal for which I am grateful. Many of the questions that arise are, of course, still unanswerable, but what follows may at least explain why. For afflicted families looking back I hope a greater understanding may help them to come to terms with the past. For those starting out, or currently grappling with the difficulties of treatment, I hope they will gain as much insight into their predicament as possible. I also hope anyone else who wishes to learn more about these dreadful diseases will be able to do so.

J. S. L.

*Sheffield*
1994

# the**facts**

## CONTENTS

# Contents

# 1

# How it all starts

## William and Mary

William Smith is 3 years old, the second child of an insurance broker and a teacher. He lives on a modern housing estate on the outskirts of a small northern industrial town. He has an older sister, Lucy, aged 5. It is summer.

One day his leg starts to ache. It hurts when he runs around, so he sits grumpily playing with his toys and half watching the television. He cries, but can be distracted and consoled. The ache eases, and his mother, who had realized something was wrong, relaxes. The normal bedtime battle reassures her.

That weekend, William's grandmother comes to visit. She lives in Kent, and has not seen the family for 6 months. She comments that William is looking rather pasty and doesn't seem quite as bright as usual. The remark is dismissed by her daughter without reply, but a tiny seed of unease, planted a few days earlier, begins to germinate. He *wasn't* quite himself, it was true. And he cries again this morning, saying his legs hurt again.

All is well for the next 2 days, but on Wednesday morning William is not awake at the usual time, cries on being woken, and is reluctant to get up. When he is coaxed out of bed, he is miserable and his mother notices he is limping. She phones the family doctor and makes an appointment to take William to the surgery the following day. By then he feels better again; the doctor examines him and reassures his mother that there is nothing to find, but agrees he looks pale and prescribes a bottle of iron tonic.

The intermittent leg pains persist and become more frequent over the next few days, and one of his mother's friends remarks on William's pallor. He is taken back to the family doctor, who looks puzzled and decides to send him to the local district hospital for a blood test 'just to be on the safe side'. Meanwhile his mother should carry on with the iron tonic and bring him back in a week for a further check and the result of the blood test.

Although the staff at the hospital are very pleasant, William screams when his blood sample is taken, and his mother, already very worried by the whole business, leaves distraught with the inconsolable toddler. They go home.

At 5 o'clock the same evening the family doctor calls to say that he has some news and wants to come round to discuss it. He sounds evasive. He will be round after surgery at about 7 o'clock. By this time William's mother is tearful and telephones her husband. He senses her distress and leaves for home immediately. They pace about the kitchen. 'I don't *know* what it is; it must be something serious, but he wouldn't say.'

The doctor arrives. He is ill at ease, and asks Mr and Mrs Smith to sit down, first suggesting that Lucy take William to watch television. He clears his throat. 'I had a call from the laboratory about William's blood test. It seems he is very anaemic. They say that he needs to go into hospital for further tests to find out why.' He pauses. 'Do they have any idea?' asks William's father. 'I must be honest with you. It looks as though he might have leukaemia.'

There is a silence. The parents stare at the doctor, who eventually carries on, 'I'm afraid William needs to go into hospital tomorrow morning at the latest. I have spoken to the paediatric team there and they are expecting him at 9 o'clock. But please don't worry unnecessarily—we don't know for certain that it is leukaemia, and even if it is treatment is usually successful these days.' William's mother starts crying silently and his father struggles to maintain composure. Neither makes any comment but they grip each other's hands. At this point William and Lucy burst in arguing noisily. They look at the three adults, fall silent, and shuffle out again. The doctor takes a deep breath. 'Any questions?'

William's father asks in a shaky voice if the doctor is certain about leukaemia and is told he is, as far as is possible at that stage. The doctor rises to leave. William's mother looks up and whispers the only words she has uttered in the whole interview. 'He will be all right, won't he?' The doctor mutters bland reassurance and avoids her direct gaze. He shakes the father's hand and leaves.

Hasty arrangements are made for Lucy to stay at a friend's house, and William and his parents make an early start for the local hospital the next morning. William is irritable and his legs are hurting. He cannot understand why his mother and father are so upset, but it is very clear that they are. Half-hearted attempts are made to appease him, and his mother hugs him. They drive in silence.

They have trouble parking at the hospital. Eventually they find a space several blocks away from the paediatric wing behind the boiler house. William's father carries him in his arms, and after a couple of wrong turns they find some doors painted with Snow White and Pluto and go in. A young nurse welcomes them and takes them to a day room with toys scattered around. William finds some farm animals to play with while the nurse takes the family details. Half an hour later a casually dressed young woman with a stethoscope round her neck and a brightly painted name badge ('Nina') comes to see them, introduces herself as 'the SHO' and carefully takes notes of William's story while he plays. Then she talks to William who eyes her warily and starts to cry as she lifts him on to his mother's lap. He grizzles while he is examined, then stays on his mother's lap, sucking his thumb.

Nina explains that there is a need to check the blood count and do one or two other tests before William's parents can be told anything further. They go to another room followed by a nurse with a trolley, and William screams for the whole 5 minutes it takes to put a small plastic tube into a vein in his wrist and collect some blood samples. The tube is anchored with tape and connected to a plastic bag of clear fluid hung upside down on a metal stand. The fluid then very slowly drips into the vein and the sweating William calms down when he and his parents go back to the day room. He falls asleep on his mother's lap. Another 2 hours pass.

A slightly harassed looking lady then appears and introduces herself as Dr Nugent, the consultant paediatrician. All the tension floods back into William's mother's face. The Smiths are told that the probability of William having leukaemia of some sort is about 95 per cent, but to be certain he will have to have his bone marrow examined. Because the diagnosis of leukaemia in children and the planning of treatment need to be done in specialist centres, William will have to be transferred to another hospital 40 miles away. But before he goes he will need a blood transfusion because his haemoglobin is only 30 per cent of what it should be. The transfer is arranged for the next day. Mrs Smith eats nothing and begins to look as if she, too, could benefit from a blood transfusion as she watches the red liquid slowly dripping into William's wrist.

The following morning William is given no breakfast and he and his mother are taken by ambulance to the University Hospital while Mr Smith follows in the family car. They are expected, greeted by the nurse in charge, and shown to a bed in a room with three others. Two are unoccupied, and one contains an unconcerned girl of about Lucy's age busy with a colouring book and some felt-tipped pens. An unremarkable scene except for two things. One is that she is completely bald. The other is that she has a complicated looking system of plastic tubing coming out of her pyjamas and attached by the side of the bed to a variety of plastic bags hung on a stainless steel stand with two flashing electronic gadgets bolted on to it. A man, presumably her father, sits nearby reading the sports page of the newspaper. He smiles. 'Hello. You must be the new patient. We heard one was coming.'

Family details are again taken by a nurse, and a short while later a Nina-like SHO introduces herself as one of the doctors from the paediatric oncology team. A pinker and now less fractious William is carefully re-examined. Mr and Mrs Smith are told that William will have a chest X-ray and then go to the operating theatre anaesthetic room. There he will be put to sleep and have some samples of bone marrow taken along with some spinal fluid from a lumbar puncture. The Smiths nod, they feel numbed, still not being quite sure what bone marrow looks like or how samples of it are taken, and not being clear why a lumbar puncture is necessary. The young doctor explains that no cutting is involved, bone marrow is obtained by a needle pushed into the hip bone. The lumbar puncture is needed to see if the leukaemia (presuming now that William definitely has leukaemia) has spread to the brain and spinal cord. The parents sign the consent form for the procedures and the anaesthetic. A more senior doctor then comes to the bedside and explains that the diagnosis of leukaemia is not in much doubt, but that the exact type and extent of the disease must be determined. An hour or two after the initial tests have been done he should be in a position to sit down with the Smiths and go into more detail about what William has and what will be done about it.

A nurse then takes the Smiths to the X-ray department. William doesn't want to co-operate, but is coaxed skilfully through the procedure by a young woman in a white uniform. The result is judged to be normal, and, after a short wait, the call comes to take the patient down to the operating suite. Mrs Smith goes with William and the nurse, Mr Smith waits on the ward.

Suspiciously eyeing the approaching doctor clad in strange green pyjamas from the vantage point of his mother's lap, William is persuaded to breathe from the end of a tube held in the anaesthetist's cupped hand. He falls asleep, lolls over, and is gently lifted on to the nearby trolley. Mrs Smith wipes away some fresh tears and is taken back to the ward by the nurse. Both parents then wait apprehensively.

An hour later William is back on the ward and wide awake. He is enjoying a drink of orange juice and a piece of buttered toast. His parents relax slightly and have a cup of tea, chatting with the nurses. Another 2 hours pass, at which stage the nurse in charge tells the Smiths that the consultant is ready to see them. William is entertained by a nursery nurse with a seemingly endless variety of toys as his parents go to a quiet office where they sit down with the consultant, the nurse from the ward, and a non-uniformed woman who is introduced as the Malcolm Sargent social worker. They prepare themselves for the worst.

The consultant explains that any remaining doubt about William having leukaemia has been dispelled, that he definitely has the disease, and that it is most probably the acute lymphoblastic variety. This is, as far as possible, good news in that the outlook for childhood lymphoblastic leukaemia is optimistic with an odds-on chance of complete cure. At that point the Smiths take each other's hands and breathe out with relief. The doctor goes on to explain that the treatment will last 2 years, that William will be kept in for most of the next 4–8 weeks while the disease is brought under control. After that Dr Nugent will be able to treat him as an out-patient at their local hospital with only occasional visits to University Hospital for special modules of chemotherapy. While most children respond satisfactorily to treatment, some do not, and if the disease returns the chances of eventual cure become very much smaller.

There is a long discussion about what leukaemia is, how it affects the blood, what treatment involves, how it works, and what the side-effects might be. The Smiths are in a daze. It is just 72 hours since William had his blood test in the local hospital, and their world has been turned upside down. The only thing they remember is that he should be cured and that his hair will probably fall out for a few months—like the little girl in the bed opposite.

There is talk of nationwide clinical trials in childhood leukaemia and of a current study for which William is eligible. They are asked to agree to let William enter the trial and they do so, not because (despite a detailed explanation) they yet fully understand the rationale and structure of the trial (though they will), but because they understand that such trials are the reason for past progress. And that they represent the best available option for treatment.

A sinister note creeps in when it is explained that not all the test results are yet available and that very occasionally surprise findings can put children into categories with a higher risk of a poor treatment response. The moment passes. The Smiths are asked if they have any questions. Mrs Smith struggles to gather her bruised thoughts together. 'Why did he ... how did he ... I mean, should we have *known*? Was it something we did?' No, it was not anything the parents had done or not done, and the cause is unknown. No other questions can be thought of. The meeting ends on a positive note with the parents being encouraged to take things one day at a time while maintaining an attitude of cautious optimism. They go back to see how William is.

Over the next few days things settle into a pattern. Mr Smith goes home to be with Lucy and her grandmother (who has come to stay), spending afternoons and evenings at the hospital, and Mrs Smith stays in the hospital with William whose treatment begins with tablets and injections. It is hard to decide which of these is more of a battle, but the nurses are very good at both.

Mrs Smith has time to meet other parents and children. The little girl in the bed opposite has a rare bone cancer for which part of the treatment is repeated courses of hospital-based chemotherapy. There are six other patients with leukaemia on the ward. One, a little girl of 4, had presented like William a week before with a very similar story. Two older children are in with presumed infections—high temperatures after a particularly 'heavy' phase of treatment—and are being given intravenous antibiotics and transfusions of things called platelets. They apparently have a different type of leukaemia from William. Their parents say the chances of eventual cure are only 50:50 at best. One is 14, and hates being in hospital. She knows she has leukaemia and does not want to talk about it.

One boy has just had a bone marrow transplant from his younger sister. He has had leukaemia for 4 years, but his first course of treatment did not get rid of it. He relapsed 12 months after it was finished. He hopes the transplant will do the job second time around. He is being nursed in an isolation cubicle but looks very well. He glumly tells Mrs Smith through the open door that he is going to have to live with girl's blood from now on. Two other children have a similar disease to William and have been on treatment for around 5 months. They are having what the nurses call 'intensification' treatment. They seem well. Mrs Smith notices that they are having their drugs dripped or injected into a rubbery white tube which disappears into the skin on the front of their chests. The other end of the tube, she has been told, is in a big vein in the chest, and the beauty of it is that children can be plugged and unplugged on to drips without needles in the hands or feet.

William does well. A week after starting treatment his bone marrow is almost clear of leukaemia, and 4 weeks later he is completely back to normal health ('in complete remission' his parents are told). He has a central venous catheter sticking out of his chest of which he is very proud. He goes home for a few days. Meanwhile another problem for the ward team is brewing.

It is now August. Mary O'Callaghan is 8. She is on holiday with her mother, father, and sister in the Yorkshire Dales. Unusually (for her) she complains about walking and climbing hills. She keeps stopping to get her breath back and complains that she doesn't feel well. When she gets home, her mother notices that she has several bruises on her legs and a large one on her back that cannot be explained. There are also some pin-point purple spots over her neck and upper arms. She looks unwell, and is listless, complaining of a headache. A nosebleed starts for no apparent reason and takes over an hour to stop. She feels hot. She is taken to morning surgery and her family doctor takes one look at her and arranges for her urgent admission to the local hospital. There she has a blood test, a short while later a blood transfusion is started, and she is transferred within 6 hours to the same ward as William in the University Hospital the day after he went home.

By the time she arrives, she is very hot, not aware of what is going on, rolling her head from side to side and moaning. More blood tests are done, and a transfusion of platelets is given, together with some intravenous antibiotics. A special X-ray scan of her head is performed, and a bone marrow test done under local anaesthetic because the doctors do not feel she is fit enough to be put to sleep. The procedure does not bother her; indeed, she does not seem to feel it at all.

The consultant speaks to Mary's parents shortly after the scan and bone marrow test. He explains that Mary apparently has acute myeloid leukaemia, unusual for a child of her age, and that she has had a small bleed into her brain. There is also the possibility that she has an infection with bacteria in her bloodstream (*septicaemia*, he called it) and she is, in short, fighting for her life.

Over the next 24 hours, Mary improves. Her temperature comes down, and she becomes more aware of her surroundings, though she is still very ill. The next day she is better still and the subject of clinical trials is raised. Mary's parents are still confused and struggling to adapt. They listen to the careful explanation of the nature of the current nationwide study for acute myeloid leukaemia for which Mary is eligible and agree that she can be entered into it. Like William's parents, they don't (yet) fully understand, but appreciate the need for an urgent decision so that treatment can begin. After a small operation to put in a central venous catheter, Mary then starts intravenous chemotherapy for the leukaemia. This initially makes her vomit. Further drugs are given to stop her being sick. The platelet transfusions and antibiotics continue unabated, and over the next few days slow progress is made.

The first course of chemotherapy finishes after 10 days, and, though weak and exhausted, Mary gradually becomes more like her normal self again. Three weeks later she is up and about and a further bone marrow examination shows that she is in remission.

# What can be learnt from these stories?

William Smith and Mary O'Callaghan do not exist. Their stories are simply descriptive examples of the initial experiences that children discovered to have leukaemia and their parents might have to go through. It is, of course, impossible to describe a 'typical' experience, as no two families and no two cases of leukaemia are alike, but the narrative perhaps indicates the sort of ordeal that many of them have to suffer.

To help parents like the Smiths and the O'Callaghans understand more about the problems their children face, this book is an attempt to explain simply what leukaemia is and how it is treated. Before that there is an important section dealing with cells, cancer, the blood, and bone marrow. Some parts may be difficult to understand for those with no scientific background, but please do not skip over them because the effort will be rewarded by better comprehension of the subsequent sections of the book.

For those who read no further, please remember the following point. Childhood leukaemia is a rare disease, and often starts (as in the case of William and Mary) with vague and non-specific symptoms that could be due to a huge number of trivial disorders. If one could imagine 25 000 children of all ages filling a football stadium, during any one year hundreds will look pale, complain of aches and pains, or refuse to climb hills. Only one will develop leukaemia.

# 2 Cells, genes, and cancer

To appreciate how leukaemia causes the problems it does, and what treatment is designed to achieve, first it is helpful to understand what a cell is, what genes are, and what cancer is.

## What cells are

All living organisms capable of independent existence are composed of one or more 'cells' which are minute individual chemical factories. Bacteria consist of a single cell. Human beings contain around 70 000 billion which differ in function and appearance depending on where in the body they are. They cling together to form *tissues* such as skin, bone, and muscle, and *organs* such as lungs, liver, and kidneys. Cells from the kidneys look quite different from those from the lung but they can all be imagined as tiny independent capsules of diverse appearance which have certain fundamental features in common. They vary in size, but are far too small to see with the naked eye. The largest in humans are around 0.005 nanolitres, which means that five to six million would fit inside an average sized raindrop.

A 'typical' human cell, cut in two, magnified several thousand times, and looked at as a two-dimensional image might look rather like a fried egg. The white of the egg would be the *cytoplasm* (*cyto* = cell, *plasm* = fluid), which contains a multitude of assorted chemicals busy reacting with each other and neighbouring cells through the *cell membrane*, the flexible bag-like structure that contains the cell contents. The yolk would represent the *nucleus*, the heart of the cell that contains the code, rather like a computer programme, enabling it to carry out its day-to-day tasks and to reproduce itself.

The programme controlling the cell is contained in a chemical called deoxyribonucleic acid (DNA). DNA is similar to a tightly coiled and very long piece of computer tape that carries masses of unique information in simple coded form. Individual bits or strips of that information are known as *genes*. Genes dictate the chemical activity of the cell. They fall into the two broad categories of 'housekeeping' genes that are needed in virtually all cells, and 'specialist' genes that are only active in certain cells (see below).

## How cells multiply

Cells need to reproduce to grow in number or replace those that naturally die off. They do this by dividing in a process known as *mitosis*. During mitosis the DNA in the nucleus condenses and packs itself into 23 pairs of identical sausage-shaped chunks of DNA called 'chromosomes'. These then replicate themselves and the cell cleaves in two with each daughter cell having 23 identical pairs of chromosomes. The process of mitosis is itself controlled by housekeeping genes, functioning rather like traffic lights, telling the cell to stop or to proceed with division.

All the genes that a person possesses are carried in the DNA of each cell of the body—in other words the blueprint for creating a complete new individual exists (for example) in the cells of the nose, the eyes, the liver, and the bone marrow. To take a cell from, say, the liver and make it grow into a complete new individual would create an exact copy of the same person—a clone. This is not yet possible in humans but has been achieved in a sheep, the famous Dolly, who is a carbon copy, having been grown from a single cell from the udder of another sheep. The reason it is so difficult to create a clone is that in any one cell from a mature animal only a tiny number of the genes are active. Most are switched off. What switches genes on or off is complicated and far from completely understood. It is of vital importance in understanding cancer, however.

## How cells come to differ from each other

The human egg and sperm are produced from cells in a process slightly but importantly different from mitosis where each ends up containing only one of the two pairs of chromosomes—i.e. 23 rather than 46 in all. They then fuse to produce a single cell with the usual 46, half from each parent. That single cell divides and eventually becomes a whole new individual, but the cells that derive from it develop widely different functions and appearances—a process known as *differentiation*. Some cells develop into lungs, some into liver, some into brain and spinal cord, some into bone, and so on. This is achieved by specialist genes being switched on, and the rest suppressed.

## Production control: what makes cells divide

Demand for new cells depends on their life span and whether the individual is increasing in size—as all children are, of course. A newborn baby will undergo a four-fold increase in length and gain up to 20 times his or her birth weight before reaching adulthood, gathering some 60 000 billion extra cells along the way. Not only will the extra cells have to be produced, but those that die during childhood will have to be replaced. Some cells live a very long time (such as brain cells, some of which last a lifetime) and some have a very short life (such as some of the cells in the blood, which may last a matter of hours or days). The process of cell division, which allows for growth and replacement (in children) and for replacement and repair (in adults) obviously requires tight control. Overproduction can result in abnormal accumulation or the formation of *tumours* (*tumour* = swelling, lump; often cancerous, see below), and underproduction can result in dwarfism or organ failure.

The control systems are normally extraordinarily efficient. Bone marrow is mind-boggling as will become apparent in the next chapter. To maintain the healthy status quo of the blood by replacing natural loss, some 5 million marrow cells are produced every second of every day for the entire life span of a human being. The consequence of too many divisions is sticky thick blood that will not circulate properly, and too few will cause anaemia, liability to infection, and abnormal bleeding. The signal for cells to proceed with division is complicated but dependent upon a variety of blood-borne chemicals that are produced in various bio-feedback processes in a way analogous to thermostatic control of temperature. Too many blood cells, and the signal to go fades. Too few, and the signal to go becomes louder. The chemicals that carry the signals are variously referred to as 'hormones', 'growth factors' or 'cytokines' (*cyto* = cell, *kinesis* = motion). Different types are produced in different organs and they circulate in the bloodstream.

## How cells die

Cells can be killed unnaturally if they are physically damaged (burnt, for example), or starved of oxygen, whereupon they disintegrate and spew out their contents in a process known as *necrosis* (*necros* = death). Heart muscle cells suffer this fate during a coronary thrombosis. The more common programmed death of cells at the end of their natural life span is rather different. It is an orderly process under the control of housekeeping genes, and is a much less messy process. It involves the stepwise shutdown of cell activity and the neat parcelling of cell contents for tidy disposal by the body's refuse collection systems. This auto-destructive process is called *apoptosis*, a term that is derived from the mechanism of falling leaves.

## What can go wrong with reproduction and cell death?

When a cell divides it replicates its DNA and the function of the two daughter cells depends on the accuracy of the copies. If, during the process of mitosis, the DNA becomes corrupted, some of the genes in the cells concerned will malfunction. This may not matter if they are liver genes in a kidney cell, for example, because they would not be switched on anyway, but the problem could be fatal for a cell if it involved housekeeping genes. In such circumstances the cell would normally undergo apoptosis, but the damaged genes could also include those controlling programmed self-destruction. In this event the end result just might be survival of a cell with corrupted housekeeping genes. Such a cell might, in turn, be deaf to the stop/go chemical signals needed to regulate cell growth. It would then reproduce (clone) itself in a similarly corrupted state and do so repeatedly out of normal control. This is how cancers can begin.

# Cancer

The name 'cancer' is probably derived from the old word *canker*, an 'eating, spreading sore or ulcer'. Others believe it to be from the Crab of the Zodiac, a creeping and nibbling creature. The former seems more likely. Whatever its source, it is now a collective term for diseases that have in common the uncontrolled clonal growth of genetically corrupted cells. They usually arise in a single organ. Mostly they grow in solid lumps. When easily visible (such as on the skin) they can be spotted at an early stage. When they are invisible (such as in the lung) they can become quite large before they are detected. Cancers that grow rapidly and have a tendency to spread, or that rapidly recur if removed, are called *malignant*. Those that grow slowly, do not spread, and can easily be removed are called *benign*.

What makes a cell malignant or benign is how it behaves in terms of its rate of growth and how it relates to its immediate neighbours and other organs in the body in terms of the chemicals it produces. These characteristics are, in turn, dependent on the nature and extent of the genetic corruption that made the cell cancerous in the first place. Unless successfully treated, malignant cancers are lethal through interference with the function of vital organs such as the liver, lungs, or bone marrow as they grow and spread around the body, and also due to the demands they place on the body's energy requirements, causing wasting and debility.

All cancers are due to genetic corruption somehow acquired during the process of normal cell division but this is not to say that they are directly inherited diseases. Genes in cells of the rest of the body of patients with cancer are normal. It is only the genes in the cancer cells that are abnormal. Much research is currently centred in understanding the exact nature of the genetic corruption in cancer, and certain genes seem to be more regularly involved than others.

Some are known to be involved in stop/go signalling for cell division and in their abnormal forms are sometimes referred to as *oncogenes* (*onco* = tumour). Others, normally involved in facilitating the process of apoptosis in damaged or elderly cells, fail when damaged and are called *tumour suppressor genes*. Tumour suppressor genes are of particular interest because rare families where there is an inherited defect in one of the two copies of one of these genes (we inherit two copies of nearly all our genes, one from mother, one from father) show a predisposition to certain types of cancer.

Some other cancer-predisposing genes can also be inherited, giving rise to an increased risk of breast cancer, for example, and there are some rare inherited conditions that increase the risk of leukaemia (see Chapter 14), but these only explain a tiny fraction of the total number of cases. There is much to learn about the genetics of cancer.

## Who gets cancer?

Cancers can arise at any age, though they are much more common in adults, and the risk of developing one rises with age. In the United Kingdom, only one child in 8000 will develop cancer each year. For men, this figure rises to one in 1000 for 40-year-olds, one in 100 for 60-year-olds, and one in 40 for 80-year-olds. This pattern is easy to understand if the risk of malignant DNA corruption is related to the cumulative number of cell divisions in an individual. Obviously cancer is not purely a random event and other factors such as smoking and an inherited predisposition play their part, but increasing age is a major risk factor.

Leukaemia of one type or another is the commonest childhood malignant disease forming some 30 per cent of all children's cancers. In 60-year-olds the equivalent figure is nearer 2 per cent, but because of the high incidence of other cancers in late adulthood, three times more sexagenarians will develop leukaemia.

Leukaemia is not a single cancer but a group of diseases representing malignant clones arising in developing blood cells. These cells, and the bone marrow where most of them develop, are described in the next two chapters.

# 3 Blood: what it is and what it does

Blood has always fascinated man from the earliest recorded human activities. It has been accorded mystical properties, been regarded as the seat of the soul, and still to this day people speak of 'life blood' when literally meaning the essence of life.

The truth is more mundane. Blood is simply a chemical soup with components made elsewhere floating around in it. Unlike organs such as the lungs, liver, kidneys, or bowel, it is not even a self-maintaining tissue with the capacity for renewal or repair. The cells of the blood are actually made in the bone marrow or the lymphatic system and it is a cancer of those organ systems rather than the blood itself that gives rise to leukaemia. So to say, as most do, that leukaemia is cancer of the blood is not quite technically correct.

The familiar sticky red fluid circulates round the body in a system of flexible branching pipes (*blood vessels* forming a *vascular* system). It is fundamentally a transport mechanism carrying important cells and chemicals from one part of the body to another. These may be waste products *en route* to the kidneys, hormones or growth factors produced in one organ to influence the activity of another, or, vitally and most importantly, oxygen from the lungs destined for all cells in the body. The cells that travel around have various different jobs as described below. The blood is kept circulating by the heart, which is not the seat of emotion (that's the brain) but merely a sophisticated pump.

Blood comprises around 7 per cent of the total weight of the body, and a fully grown man will have around 5 litres in his circulation (nearly 9 pints). A 'drop of blood', as referred to in this chapter, is the amount that might fall to the floor from a cut finger, and is calculated to be 0.000033 of a litre or 0.00006 pints.

If a small test-tube full of blood is taken, prevented from clotting, and then left to settle, it will separate out into a clear straw-coloured

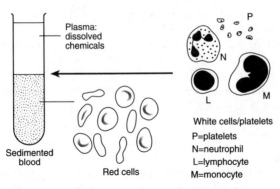

**Figure 1.** Constituents of normal blood with drawings of cells magnified 1000 times.

top half—the *plasma*—and a dark-red bottom half—the red cells. In between will be a fine white band, called the 'buffy coat', which contains the white cells of various types (collectively called *leucocytes*: *leuco* = white, *cyto* = cell), and a third type of small cells called *platelets* (Fig. 1).

## Plasma

In health, just over half of the total quantity of blood is the clear, straw-coloured fluid called plasma. In it is dissolved a multitude of complex and important chemicals, some only found in plasma and there for a specific purpose, some found in all body fluids, and some simply hitching a ride from one part of the body to another. If plasma is separated from blood and left to stand without special treatment it will clot into jelly, or *coagulate*. The fluid that can be poured off the clot at that stage is called *serum*. It contains all the same things as plasma apart from the chemicals involved in blood clotting.

## Blood cells

Some 40–45 per cent of the volume of blood is accounted for by cells, small flexible bags which form individual units with their own internal environment under tight biochemical control (see Chapter 2). Older texts refer to the blood cells as *corpuscles*, but as the term is not used for cells in other body tissues, it is perhaps illogical to retain it just for use when referring to blood.

Blood cells are of three basic types. By far the most numerous are the red cells, which give blood its characteristic colour. The next most numerous are the tiny *platelets*, and finally the least frequent cells, though the most important as far as leukaemia is concerned, the white cells, or *leucocytes*. Each will be considered in turn.

## Red cells

The red cells of the blood are also known as *erythrocytes* (*erythro* = red, *cyte* = cell). Their sole function is to provide a transport vehicle for a vital bright-red chemical called *haemoglobin* (see below). They are small, round, and shaped roughly like a squash ball squeezed firmly between finger and thumb—a flattened sphere with large dimples opposite each other. Each drop of blood from a healthy child (or adult) will contain over 150 million red cells. They are produced in the bone marrow, and have a finite life span. When exhausted, they die and are replaced. The turnover is finely balanced in health, so that the number of red cells, and the amount of haemoglobin they contain, is kept within a fairly narrow range. The life span of a red cell is 3–4 months, so the loss and replacement each day is of the order of 1 per cent of the total. This means that the bone marrow has to produce some three million red cells every second to keep pace with natural loss.

*Haemoglobin* (*haemo* = blood, *globin* = a type of protein) is a chemical compound that has the capacity to take hold of oxygen where there is plenty in the immediate vicinity, and then to let go of it again when there is not. This is essential, because all cells in the body use oxygen to fuel the chemical reactions that keep them alive.

The equivalent of the whole blood volume (5 litres in an adult) goes through the heart every 60 seconds to keep the process of oxygen transport humming along at breakneck speed, but various things can go wrong with the system. If the number of red cells, or the amount of haemoglobin they contain, becomes reduced below normal, the resulting state is called *anaemia*, a word that literally means 'no blood'.

Patients with anaemia look pale. This is because the amount of haemoglobin in the blood is reduced. But pallor is not always due to anaemia. People can look pale for other reasons. Some have a naturally sallow complexion. Truly anaemic patients with very low amounts of haemoglobin in the circulation (20 per cent of average normal) will have a waxen appearance and (tellingly) very pale lips.

## Platelets

The least visible, least well-known, but vitally important small blood cells called platelets were the last blood cells to be discovered. They are around a fifth to a quarter the size of red cells, but are colourless and contain no pigment. It was not until 1868 that they were discovered to have a function in controlling bleeding.

The name 'platelet' was derived from the original German 'Blutplättchen' (*Blut* = blood, *Plättchen* = plate), a term coined by a writer of the time who fancied that the small discus-shaped cells he was describing looked like small plates.

They are formed in the bone marrow from huge cells called *megakaryocytes* (*mega* = great, *karyon* = nucleus, *cyte* = cell) in a unique process not the result of mitosis but of bits of the cell cytoplasm breaking off, or budding, and floating away as individual platelets. Each drop of blood from a healthy individual will contain some 7–10 million. They live, unless called for active service, for 1–2 weeks, so some 10 per cent are lost through reaching the end of their natural life each day. On that basis they need to be replaced at the rate of around one and a half million every second, about half the rate of red cells.

The role of platelets is to stop bleeding and to maintain the circulation in good shape. They have the capacity to stick together (aggregate) to plug small holes appearing anywhere in blood vessels.

Platelet numbers can fall for two basic reasons; either insufficient are being produced, or the survival of those produced is shortened by rapid consumption (or a combination of both). Numbers have to fall to 10 per cent of average normal or less before any outward effects will be noticed, but eventually excessive bruising and tiny purple spots under the skin will appear. These are pin-point bleeds called *petechiae*. The presence of multiple petechiae is referred to as a *purpura* (purple skin discoloration). A low platelet count is called *thrombocytopenia* (*thrombocytes* = an alternative name for platelets, *penia* = lack of).

## White cells

White cells in the blood are, like platelets, colourless. If they are collected in large enough quantities, separated from the red cells, and packed together, they have a milky opalescent appearance. There are two basic types with fundamentally different tasks; the granulocytes/ monocytes and the lymphocytes. Each will be considered in turn.

## Granulocytes and monocytes

These cell types are really first cousins, both being derived from the same ancestral cells in the bone marrow (see Chapter 4).

*Granulocytes* are so-called because they have speckled granules in the cytoplasm when studied with a microscope. They consist of three subtypes, *neutrophils*, *eosinophils*, and *basophils*. These names refer to their staining pattern with the dyes used to make them visible under the microscope.

Each drop of healthy blood will contain 130–140 000 neutrophils—slightly less in very young babies. They are, like many of the blood cells, destined to die rather than reproduce, but they leave the circulation and wriggle into the confined spaces between cells of other tissues before perishing. Their true life span is thus not easy to measure, but it is likely that the bone marrow has to pump out some 120 000 each second to maintain average numbers for an adult.

Neutrophils are true scavengers. They are the refuse men of the bloodstream and tissues. They have the capacity to engulf and ingest particles, living (such as bacteria) or dead (such as cell debris) in a process known as *phagocytosis* (*phago* = eating). For this reason they are also known as phagocytes, but share this non-exclusive title with other cells derived from their first cousins the monocytes (see below). They play a vital role in the process of *inflammation*, the response of the body to injury or invasion characterized by heat, swelling, redness, and pain. They phagocytose micro-organisms and kill them by powerful enzyme attack. By piling into the site of infection (a boil or tooth abscess would be a good example) they help to prevent it from spreading and aid the process of healing. In patients with other than trivial bacterial infections, the blood neutrophils can increase in number up to five- or six-fold. In short, they are invaluable.

Complete *neutropenia* (lack of neutrophils) is a life-threatening state. While powerful injected antibiotics can kill bacteria and so compensate to some extent, prolonged and total absence of neutrophils is invariably fatal in the end. Fortunately, there is a great difference between *no* neutrophils and a *greatly reduced number*. Just two to five per cent of average normal numbers are enough to avoid serious difficulties, and 20 per cent will not be associated with any special problems at all.

Eosinophils look much like neutrophils, but are not so numerous. A drop of blood will contain only 7000 or so. Their numbers increase in a variety of disorders, chiefly allergic reactions (asthma, for example), or invasive parasitic infections (tapeworms, for example). They have no obvious vital function.

Basophils are the rarest and the least understood leucocytes. They are similar in appearance to neutrophils until stained with Romanowsky dyes, when they appear a deep, dense purple. There are usually no more than 2000 in each drop of blood and may be considerably less. What they do is not clear but they do not seem to be particularly important.

*Monocytes* belong to the same family as granulocytes but look rather different. They have no granules in the cytoplasm. They are the biggest cells in the blood, being up to three times the size of red cells and twice the size of neutrophils. A drop of blood will contain 30–40 000.

Their time in the circulation (usually short, perhaps of the order of 12–24 hours) is a transitional phase as they progress to tissues outside the bloodstream. There they mature further and change their appearance to become large scavengers called *macrophages* (*macro* = large, *phago* = eating), functioning as heavy duty refuse disposal units. They are less efficient and less important than neutrophils.

## Lymphocytes

Lymphocytes are the second most numerous type of white cell in the blood of adults, and the most numerous in the blood of children up to the age of about 4 years, after which their circulating numbers subside. They are so-called because they also heavily populate the *lymphatic system*, a body-wide arrangement of tiny drainage channels. The fluid in these drains (*lymph*) is not pumped by the heart, but is intermittently squeezed along as the body moves and muscles in the arms and legs contract. The purpose of having a drainage system of this sort is to return material lying outside cells and outside the bloodstream back to the blood.

Not surprisingly, lymph picks up its fair share of rubbish. Like most drainage and sewage networks, it has a filtration system, and the lymphatic vessels pass through small oval or bean-shaped bodies called *lymph nodes* or *lymphatic glands*. These vary in size from a pea to a small plum. They are packed with lymphocytes and macrophages, and the latter scavenge any refuse or micro-organisms. They can enlarge considerably when close to an infection and can become tender. Most people have suffered lumps under the angle of the jaw in association with a sore throat. These are swollen lymph nodes.

Lymphocytes populate the lymph nodes (where some of them reproduce) and roll out along the lymphatic drainage channels into the blood. They have a variable appearance and size, with the smallest being no bigger than a red cell. A drop of blood from a newborn baby may have up to half a million, falling to half that by the age of 4, and to 100 000 or less by the time adulthood is reached.

They are not all the same, nor are they even all made in the same place. Collectively they form a vital component of the body's immune system (for defence against invasion by bacteria or viruses), of which there are several distinct but interrelated parts. These parts are reflected by the main different functional types of lymphocyte of which there are two; T lymphocytes (so-called because they are associated with the thymus gland), and B lymphocytes (so-called because they are derived from the bone marrow). Their appearance may be similar under the microscope, but they have different roles in the body's defences.

In health, the proportions of the various types of lymphocyte circulating in the blood are roughly 65 per cent T cells and 25 per cent B cells. The remaining 10 per cent are a miscellany of other types, the exact function of which is still not clear. The life span of lymphocytes is very variable with some surviving many years. They tend to be created in bursts of activity when there is some immune challenge to the body such as an infection, and there is no controlled number with a regular replacement pattern, as with red cells. Most of them at any one time will not be circulating in the blood, but will be in the lymph nodes, spleen, or other tissues, such as the tonsils.

## Blood counts

Loose reference to 'blood counts' usually means a combined test to count red cells, white cells (all types), and platelets, together with a measurement of the amount of haemoglobin the blood contains. These figures are produced by sophisticated machines from a drop of blood in a few seconds. The normal values for children for the various components vary according to age.

The results are often discussed in conversation in a type of shorthand. To say, for example, that 'the haemoglobin is 7.3' actually means that the patient concerned has a blood concentration of haemoglobin of 7.3 grams per decilitre (or 73 grams per litre). Similarly, to say that the 'white count is two' means that the total of all types of white cell is $2.0 \times 10^9$ (2 000 000 000) per litre, of which the neutrophils might be, say, 50 per cent or $1 \times 10^9$ (1 000 000 000) per litre. Some confusion lingers over the now accepted use of SI (Système International) units. This system changed white counts (and platelet counts) from thousands per cubic millimetre to $10^9$ per litre, which divided the old number used by 1000. So a white count of 4000 became a white count of four, and a platelet count of 200 000 became one of 200, and so on. Some doctors and scientists still use the old system in conversation, and so, for example, refer to a neutrophil count of $1.5 \times 10^9$ per litre as '15 hundred'. To make matters worse, in the United States, SI units have been eschewed by some scientific authorities and for blood counts the cubic millimetre is still preferred. In some blood diseases, including the leukaemias, where normal counts can vary 100-fold, it is essential for everyone to be very clear exactly what they mean.

When abnormal blood counts from machines are encountered, it is usual for laboratories to examine a stained smear of blood under the microscope as well. The red cells can then be visually examined and the proportion of white cells falling into the various categories can be checked by counting 100 consecutive cells and expressing each type as a percentage of the total. This is called a *differential* white cell count, and why lymphocyte counts, for example, are sometimes referred to as so many 'per cent'. To think of cell counts in terms of percentages, however, is potentially misleading. A reduction in one cell type can lead to an increased percentage of another without any increase in numbers. It is always safer to stick to absolute numbers.

Average normal blood counts for children of different ages are given in Table 1.

**Table 1.** Average normal blood counts for children of different ages

| Age | Hb | WBC | NC | LC | Plts |
|---|---|---|---|---|---|
| Newborn | 15–24 | 10–26 | 2.5–14 | 2–7 | 150–450 |
| 6 months | 10–13 | 6–17 | 1–6 | 3–12 | 200–550 |
| 1 year | 10–13 | 6–16 | 1–8 | 3–10 | 200–550 |
| 2–6 years | 11–14 | 6–17 | 1.5–8.5 | 2–8 | 200–500 |
| 6–12 years | 11–15 | 4.5–14.5 | 1.5–8 | 1.5–5 | 180–450 |
| 12–18 boys | 12–17 | 4.5–13 | 1.5–6 | 1.5–4.5 | 180–400 |
| 12–18 girls | 12–15 | 4.5–13 | 1.5–6 | 1.5–4.5 | 180–400 |

Hb = haemoglobin, WBC = white blood cells, NC = neutrophil count,
LC = lymphocyte count, Plts = platelet count. Units are: Hb: g/dl (multiply by 10 for g/l); WBC, NC, LC, Plts: $\times 10^9$/l (multiply by 1000 for /mm³).

# 4
# Bone marrow: the blood cell factory

## What marrow is

All the cells circulating in healthy blood, except for some of the lymphocytes, are produced in the bone marrow, which is a type of seed-bed. Marrow is found inside all bones, which are hollow, even those of the ribs, skull, shoulder blade, and breastbone. If a rib were to be removed and cut in half longways, there would be a rim of hard bone on the outside and some soft red material oozing blood on the inside. If poked with a pencil, the soft red material would have a crunchy feel to it, like honey-comb or a firm meringue. Marrow consists of a loose meshwork of bony strands (which give the bone increased strength like cross-struts on scaffolding) interspersed with open caverns of blood supplied by millions of tiny pipes taking blood to and from the caverns. In little lakes of blood deep in this system blood cells are produced.

The total potential marrow space in the bones of an adult is around 3 litres (5 pints). Only a proportion, however, is used for blood cell production. That part is called 'red' marrow because of its appearance as described above. In adults, 'red' marrow is largely confined to what is called the 'axial' skeleton—the bones excluding the arms and legs. The bones of the extremities are generally not used for blood cell production, but are full of large storage cells containing oil, an energy reserve. This material is called 'yellow' marrow. In infants, because the demand for new blood cells is so great, *all* the bones are used for blood production, and there is no 'yellow' marrow. In effect, the amount of active 'red' marrow is much the same in a 3-year-old child as it is in an adult, and occupies a volume of some 1.5 litres or 2.5 pints. The amount of 'yellow' marrow gradually increases with age.

An old term for bone marrow is the Greek word *myelos* which means marrow or core. The word is no longer heard, but the prefix *myelo-* is still used widely to describe things related to the marrow. For example, it is used in the description of some developing blood cells—*myelocytes* and *promyelocytes* are names for recognizable forms of developing granulocytes—and *myelo-suppression* is used to refer to marrow function being restricted in some way. The word *myeloid* means 'marrow-like', or, more commonly by popular usage, 'like a developing granulocyte', and is sometimes used to describe cells from a patient with leukaemia to suggest that the disease comes from developing granulocytes rather than lymphocytes.

## How blood cells grow

Developing blood cells look different from their mature counterparts. The earliest recognizable forms of all the different types of blood cell are called *blasts*. Blast is derived from a Greek word meaning to sprout or germinate, and refers to a cell capable of further growth and specialization. Immature red cells are called *erythroblasts*. Immature granulocytes are called *myeloblasts*, *promyelocytes*, and *myelocytes* (with increasing degrees of maturation), immature monocytes are called *monoblasts*, and immature lymphocytes *lymphoblasts*.

Consider the following statistics. As already indicated, the demand for red cells is around three million per second (260 billion per day). The demand for platelets is some one and a half million per second (130 billion per day), and the demand for white cells (nearly all neutrophils) is of the order of 120 000 per second (10 billion per day). So the marrow, on average, produces nearly five million cells every second, or a staggering 400 billion every 24 hours. That figure is for healthy 'tickover'. In circumstances of increased demand, supply can be stepped up four- to five-fold or more to avoid shortages. Where bleeding causes loss of red cells, where there is rapid consumption of platelets (bleeding, severe infection), or where infection by bacteria temporarily greatly increases the demand for neutrophils, the marrow can cope up to a point, provided it is healthy.

## Growth factors

Cells growing in normal marrow are influenced by chemicals produced elsewhere in the body in a type of thermostatic control system.

Too few cells, and the relevant chemical concentration is increased to 'drive' the marrow to produce more. A glut of cells, and the concentration falls so production ceases. There are different chemicals that drive the different cell types. Red cells are driven by erythropoietin (*erythro* = red, *poiesis* = growth), platelets by thrombopoietin, and neutrophils not by neutropoietin (which would be logical) but a substance called granulocyte colony stimulating factor or G-CSF for short. The name comes from the laboratory experiments that led to its discovery. It was a substance that was found to promote the growth of neutrophils in culture plates outside the body where the cells grow in colonies. A closely related compound is callled GM-CSF, and this promotes the growth of both neutrophils and monocytes.

It is now possible to give all these chemicals as drugs to provide an artificial marrow drive to produce more red cells, platelets, neutrophils, or monocytes. They will only work on marrow that has the capacity to increase production, however, so if the cell production lines are shut down (see marrow failure, below) they will not have any effect. G-CSF is used to hasten marrow recovery from cancer chemotherapy in some circumstances (see Chapter 12) or occasionally following marrow transplantation.

It is easy to understand that the fine balance of supply and demand occasionally becomes disturbed. Where supply fails to meet demand (the more usual problem), shortages arise in one or more categories of blood cell, depending on the cause of the supply failure. The result is a *cytopenia* (*cyto* = cell, *penia* = lack of). Lack of neutrophils is called a *neutropenia*, lack of platelets a *thrombocytopenia* (platelets are also known as thrombocytes), and lack of all blood cells is called a *pancytopenia* (*pan* = everything). Lack of red cells could logically and precisely be called an *erythro-cytopenia*, as red cells are also known as erythrocytes, but it is more usually referred to as *anaemia* which literally means 'no blood'. This is because a great lack of red cells produces a bloodless pallor, and the condition was recognized long before blood cells were discovered.

More unusually, where supply exceeds demand, an excess of cells can be found. This circumstance implies a lack of growth regulation of the cells of the marrow, but need not always be due to a type of cancer. If a period of increased demand suddenly comes to an end, for example, the marrow might not shut down supply rapidly enough, so there will be a period of 'overshoot'.

Prolonged increased marrow output over demand is a sign of uncontrolled cell growth and usually indicates a form of cancer—one of the leukaemias. When one cell line goes out of normal control, production of others can be interfered with leading to the hallmark of all types of leukaemia—failure of normal bone marrow function.

## Bone marrow failure

When cytopenias occur, either because cells are being destroyed prematurely and the marrow cannot keep up an adequate supply, or because marrow production falters in one or more cell assembly line, the marrow fails to fulfil its role. Everyone is familiar with the concept of kidney failure, or heart failure. Bone marrow failure should be thought of in much the same way, even though the marrow is not so well defined as an anatomical organ. Failure can be partial or total and involve one cell line or more.

More common than problems with a single cell line, the marrow shows disturbances affecting *all* production systems producing a *pancytopenia*. This is for one of two basic reasons. Either there is something intrinsically wrong with the orderly procession of stem cells through intermediate forms to mature blood cells, or some external influence has interfered with the system. Put simply, either the marrow just peters out or something destroys it. Petering out and the production of blood cells just fading away is known as *hypoplastic* or *aplastic anaemia* (*hypo* = low, few; *a* = none; *plastic* = growth, development).

In children marrow output fails more commonly because the marrow itself is choked up with immature (malignant) cells derived either from one of the marrow's own production lines or appearing as unwelcome squatters from a disease site elsewhere in the body.

All childhood leukaemias can cause marrow failure in this way and that is what makes them potentially fatal diseases. Some leukaemias arise in the marrow, others arise in the lymphatic system outside marrow and move in. Infiltrating diseases other than leukaemia can occasionally cause similar problems, but they are nearly all malignant cancers, and only produce marrow failure as a late feature in their advanced stages.

In truth the effect on bone marrow function of infiltrating malignant cells is more complicated than a simple 'crowding out' of normal marrow cells. Some leukaemias produce a suppressive effect early in their development, whereas others can reach an enormous size in terms of tumour growth alongside fairly well-preserved marrow function. It is likely that different tumours produce different chemicals that directly affect the growth of nearby normal cells.

# How marrow is examined

There are two basic ways of looking at marrow. The first is to push in a needle, suck out a few drops of fluid (which is blood heavily contaminated with marrow cells), and then to smear a drop very thinly on to a microscope slide. That smear is then stained with Romanowsky dyes and examined at a magnification of around 1000-fold so that the individual cells can be seen, identified, counted, and the proportions of each type assessed. The technique is called *aspiration cytology* and provides information on the *type* of cells present and their proportions (which may be all one needs to know), but does not give a reliable view of the architecture of the marrow or the overall *number* of cells present. The latter may be important if only a few cells are obtained and there is doubt about whether a patient has marrow failure from fade-out or overgrowth. Marrows that are heavily infiltrated with leukaemia are sometimes technically very difficult to aspirate successfully and a sample adequate to make a confident diagnosis may not be obtained.

In such circumstances it is important to obtain a *trephine biopsy*. *Trephine* is a word derived from the Latin 'trepanum', a borer, and refers to a small crown saw for cutting out small pieces of bone. *Biopsy* means removing living cells or tissue.

The procedure yields a small cylindrical core of bone together with bone marrow about the length of a fingernail and the width of thin spaghetti. It is collected with a specially designed marrow coring needle with serrated teeth on the end. The specimen is then processed in chemicals and sliced extremely thinly before being stained and examined under a microscope. The technique gives a good view of the overall number of cells present, but their detailed study is not as easy as it is using aspiration cytology. The two methods are thus complementary and not alternatives. As both are painful, and as obtaining a good trephine requires some fiddling even in experienced hands, it is usual to perform marrow specimen collection from children under a general anaesthetic.

The best site for obtaining good samples of marrow from children is the hip bone of the pelvis. In adults the breastbone is commonly used if only aspiration cytology is being attempted, though that site is not suitable for use in children. In tiny babies, because of the different distribution of red marrow it is possible to obtain samples from the larger of the two bones in the lower leg (the *tibia*), and this is sometimes easier than the hip bone. It is not usually possible to get adequate trephine samples from children under 6 months of age.

In addition to simple microscopy, other tests can be performed on marrow samples. The chromosomes and genes of the cells of an aspirate can be examined. Cells can be tested with chemical reagents and put through cell-sorting machines activated by lasers to help identify their origin or lineage where this is not obvious from their appearance. Such tests, together with routine microscopy, now form the basis of the diagnosis and classification of all leukaemias.

# 5
# Leukaemia: its frequency, causes, and diagnosis

Leukaemia is a global term for a malignant growth of blood cells and so is effectively synonymous with cancer of the bone marrow. The different varieties relate to the different marrow cell types, these all having malignant counterparts. The term also embraces cancers of lymphocytes that may start in the lymphatic system and later spread to colonize the marrow.

The word literally means 'white blood' and is a Greek derivation of the original German 'Weisses Blut'. The name was coined because the only type of disease that could be recognized before the development of powerful microscopes in the latter nineteenth century was that which gradually produced very high white cell counts with increasing anaemia. This gives the blood a strange pearlescent appearance to the naked eye. The type of disease that typically does this (chronic granulocytic leukaemia—see below and Chapter 14) rarely happens in children so childhood leukaemia was not widely recognized as a problem until around the 1880s when high quality microscopy became widely available.

At that stage two different types were recognized, *acute* and *chronic* (the medical meaning of these terms is that acute diseases run a rapid course while chronic ones run a slow gradual course). The difference was obvious not only in the patients' survival—acute leukaemia sufferers seldom survived 3 months, whereas those with the much less common chronic disorders would run a longer course—but in the appearance of the leukaemic cells. Acute leukaemias were characterized by an accumulation of similarly featured immature and poorly differentiated blood cells, referred to collectively as 'blasts', whereas the chronic disorders had cells at various stages of maturation with many appearing to be fully mature. Both types were eventually fatal, as the chronic leukaemias usually evolved into a disease with the appearances of the acute variety after a variable period of time.

The acute leukaemias were also subdivided into two other broad categories. There were those that appeared to be related to lymphocytes (*acute lymphatic* or *lymphoblastic leukaemia*, commonly abbreviated to ALL), and those that were related to granulocytes (*acute myeloid* or *myeloblastic leukaemia* commonly abbreviated to AML—or alternatively ANLL meaning *acute non-lymphoblastic leukaemia*).

There were, in addition, some marrow production disorders that fell short of frank leukaemia, but which were seen in many instances to progress to the full-blown disorder after a period of time. Some had sufficiently abnormal blood or marrow to be appreciated at an early stage to be harbingers of malignancy, and went under such names as 'smouldering leukaemia' or 'pre-leukaemia'. Others were merely regarded as 'chronic refractory anaemias'. It has subsequently become apparent that many of these miscellaneous disorders show evidence of clonality, and so have the hallmark of cancer. Collectively they have become known as the *myelodysplastic* syndromes, (*myelo* = marrow; *dys* = disordered, difficult; *plastic* = growth). They are much more common in adults than children, but do occur at all ages and are considered under the broad definition of leukaemia.

Children most frequently develop acute leukaemia involving lymphocytes (ALL), a situation reversed in adults who more often have acute disease involving granulocytes (AML). Although these two broad types of leukaemia can occur at any age, there are different subvarieties that are more or less confined to infancy and the early years of childhood and others that are unusual before late adolescence and adulthood.

Chronic leukaemias are very rare in children and invariably involve granulocytes—called *chronic myeloid* or *granulocytic leukaemia* (CML or CGL). They are of two types; one more usually seen in adults—adult-type CML—and the other more rare and unique to childhood, juvenile CML. The chronic lymphocytic leukaemia frequently seen in elderly patients does not have any counterpart in children. Further details of the different varieties of chronic childhood leukaemia are given in the relevant later sections of the book.

# The frequency of childhood leukaemia

Although collectively the leukaemias are the commonest childhood cancer, making up some 30–35 per cent of the total, they are still very rare diseases. Each year, only one child in 25 000 will develop leukaemia. That translates to just 400 from the 10 million children in the whole of the UK every 12 months and means that the average family doctor in the UK may easily never see a case in the whole of his or her career.

Of the 400 new cases each year, 300 or more will be ALL of one type or another, around 80 will be AML and the tiny remainder will be a miscellany of chronic leukaemias or myelodysplastic syndromes.

# The causes of childhood leukaemia

As indicated in Chapter 2, leukaemias, like all cancers, arise because defective gene replication during cell division (mitosis) gives rise to a cell that grows out of normal control. What sets the stage for this to happen is not fully understood, but several factors may be involved and more than one in any individual case. The first thing to appreciate is that it is unlikely that there is any single factor involved in all leukaemias. In other words the cause of ALL is unlikely to be the same as that of AML. Indeed, it is unlikely that the cause of different subtypes of ALL is the same, so the question immediately becomes quite complicated.

We have a few clues to factors that might be involved in the evolution of some leukaemias, but the picture is still very blurred and we have to start by admitting that in the vast majority of cases we simply do not know what starts the disease.

## Population mixing

For the commonest type of childhood ALL it appears that there is an increased frequency in situations where there is substantial population mixing as might occur, for example, in new towns or around large industrial plants where there is a large influx of migrant workers. This has been repeatedly shown in careful studies of several such circumstances and might explain the excess of cases seen at large remote nuclear installations such as Sellafield and Dounreay. The pattern of infections encountered by children mixing with their new peers may be different in such situations and could provide an extra challenge to their immune systems (remembering that ALL is a cancer of the immune system).

The same factors may be at work to explain the apparent excess of ALL among children who are more socially isolated in their early years—notably those living in sparsely populated rural areas and those in higher socio-economic groups.

## Defective genes acquired in the womb

From studies of leukaemia arising in identical twins it is apparent that some types of ALL may have the seeds sown before birth. This in not to say that the disease is inherited—that would involve defective genes being passed from parent to child. Rather it seems that in rare instances a defect can occur in developing lymphocytes in the fetus (for reasons that are not clear) and that this directly or indirectly gives rise to leukaemia later in childhood. If one of two identical twins develops leukaemia there is an increased risk of the other twin doing the same. In the early years of childhood this risk is highest, and it dwindles as the siblings grow older. There is no increased risk to non-identical twins.

Where twins do both develop leukaemia it is virtually always exactly the same disease down to the last genetic detail, even though there may be a gap of months or years between the two developing the disease. This is taken as evidence that one fetus develops abnormal lymphocytes in the womb and transfers them to its twin by the common circulation of their shared placenta. There is usually a variable period of latency before the disease develops, occasionally years, which suggests that there may need to be a second event or factor involved before leukaemia actually develops, at least in some instances.

## Radiation

There has been much speculation about the role of environmental radiation in the cause of childhood cancer in general and leukaemia in particular. Observed clusters of cases around nuclear installations have caused huge concern, but these may have other explanations (see population mixing, above). While there is no doubt that large doses of radiation can cause leukaemia, the unusual circumstances in which this is known to happen are irrelevant to virtually all cases in childhood. Perhaps most interestingly there has been no obvious excess of leukaemia following the Chernobyl disaster—the radiation-related cancers were almost all tumours of the thyroid gland. This is because the chief environmental contaminant—radioactive iodine—is concentrated in that organ. So it presently seems highly unlikely that environmental radiation is a major factor in the cause of childhood leukaemia.

## Viruses

No types of childhood leukaemia are known to be the direct result of a virus infection. That said, viruses certainly cause leukaemia in cats and other animal species, and a rare leukaemia-related cancer of T lymphocytes of adults, seen in Japan and the Caribbean, is known to be due to a virus from the same family as the HIV (AIDS) virus. So it is quite possible for viruses to cause cancer, but despite a vigorous search, none have been implicated so far in childhood leukaemia in a direct cause-and-effect role.

## Electromagnetic fields

Why there might be an excess chance of children developing leukaemia if they live near pylons carrying high voltage national grid power cables or near to electricity sub-stations is not clear, but the suggestion was made by some studies looking for unknown causative factors. It has not been substantiated and the theory has little credence at the present time.

## Toxic chemicals

There is no known association between toxic or agricultural chemicals and childhood leukaemia, though there may be with *aplastic anaemia* (see Chapter 4). Some anti-cancer drugs can paradoxically cause a type of AML (see Chapter 10), but this is a very infrequent complication and thankfully only occurs in a tiny number of children.

# How leukaemia is diagnosed and typed

Defining and recognizing sub-varieties of childhood acute leukaemia is becoming increasingly complicated. This is because new ways of studying the disease are continually developing, and these new techniques have to be reconciled with the older ways of categorizing the various types.

There are four fundamentally different ways of looking at leukaemia in children, these being the clinical features of the disease, the microscopic appearance of the malignant cells, the chemical profile of the malignant cells, and the abnormalities of their corrupted DNA, the chromosomes and genes.

To talk of 'types' of leukaemia inevitably introduces the other most important factor that is usually taken into consideration when attempting to categorize the disease—the likelihood of a successful outcome of treatment, but that will be considered later. To make sense of all this it is easiest to consider how a new patient is assessed at the outset.

## Clinical features

Patients complain of *symptoms* such as pain or malaise and exhibit abnormal *signs* such as enlargement of the spleen or pin-point skin bleeds. The pattern of these two, together with the history (when the problem began, what symptoms came first and when, what other illnesses the child has had, what medication, and so forth) can provide valuable information. It can point the way laboratory investigation should be directed and what kind of leukaemia might be present.

Occasionally important information is gained from *imaging* techniques. These include simple X-rays of the chest and abdomen, or ultrasound scans. They are used to detect enlargement of internal organs that cannot easily be felt by simple examination. Rarely a *CT scan* or *MR scan* may be used, usually to examine the inside of the head or spinal cord. CT stands for *computerized tomography*, and is a series of X-ray pictures taken at different angles and assembled into a composite picture by a computer. MR stands for *magnetic resonance* and produces a similar type of picture to CT but uses a very strong magnetic field instead of X-rays. It is better for looking at the spinal cord.

## Laboratory tests

A simple blood count and film microscopy will confirm or greatly strengthen the suspicion that a child has leukaemia, and will prompt urgent examination of the bone marrow. A glance down a microscope at a stained marrow smear will then usually be sufficient to say whether a child has leukaemia, and to hazard a good guess whether it is ALL or AML, and possibly even whether it is a rare subtype or not. This is based on the appearance of the blast cells (known as their *morphology*, meaning their physical shape). Occasionally getting an adequate marrow sample can be technically difficult leaving continuing doubt about the diagnosis. If that happens the marrow sampling may need to be repeated.

## Special stains on bone marrow smears

Various stains that produce colours as the result of chemical reactions can be applied to malignant cells on microscope slides, though these are no longer routinely used to distinguish between ALL and AML. They are now reserved for sub-typing AML.

## Sorting cells by specially made anti-cell antibodies

Early in the 1970s leukaemic cells from children with ALL were injected into laboratory rabbits. The rabbits, recognizing the cells as 'foreign', made antibodies to them. After extracting and carefully separating out the various antibodies, it was then possible to focus on one that seemed to react just with the original ALL leukaemic cells but not with any other human body cells. This antibody was then applied to the leukaemic cells from newly diagnosed patients and reacted with most of those with ALL. Most, but not all. Patients with ALL could thus be classified as 'common' ALL if their cells reacted with the antibody, or 'other' if they did not. The antibody was said to recognize the 'CALLA' (common ALL antigen). Diseases were designated CALLA positive or negative.

In the late 1970s and 1980s a new technology appeared that allowed the relatively easy manufacture of pure antibodies to use as testing chemicals and that could be produced in laboratories without the use of animals. These are now classified by the part of the cell they recognize, and the various parts of cells defined in this way are referred to as *clusters of differentiation*, or CD for short. CALLA has become CD10, and there are now over 150 CDs, some of which are used to help recognize whether leukaemic cells are immature lymphocytes or granulocytes, and what stage of immaturity they are frozen at. Thus it is possible to classify ALL into different stages of B or T lymphocyte development and AML into different stages of granulocyte or monocyte development.

Because the use of antibodies as chemical reagents in this way is an *immunological* technique (because antibodies are normally produced by animal immune systems), the pattern of reaction of leukaemic cells with these markers is referred to as their *immunological phenotype* (from *phenomenon*), or alternatively their *immunophenotype*. The antibody reagents are tagged with light-scattering chemicals and the cells they attach to can be fed through a machine (a flow cytometer) in a stream where positivity can be detected using a laser beam. Thousands of cells can be examined very quickly, and the proportion reacting with a given antibody worked out precisely.

Sometimes cells from children with ALL will show an aberrant or unusual pattern of positivity with different antibodies. For example, cells might show immunological features of both ALL and AML, which is rather confusing. Called *lineage infidelity*, a mixture of cell markers usually indicates that the leukaemia in question may be arising in a very early or primitive cell, and such diseases may run a different course.

## The chromosomes in leukaemic cells

As described in Chapter 2, normal human cells have 46 chromosomes in two matching sets of 23, and these contain the entire genetic information for a given individual in the form of DNA. In malignant tumours, a *clone* of cells (the progeny of a single rogue cell) develops and these aberrant cells have an acquired abnormality in their DNA which may or may not be obvious when the chromosomes are examined under a microscope. Once acquired, such abnormalities are carried through successive generations of the cells. The sort of abnormalities that might arise include abnormal numbers (more or less than the usual 46) or rearrangements where bits of one chromosome have broken off and become attached to another. The pattern of abnormalities may be apparently random, or highly specific for a certain type of cancer or leukaemia.

Not only can the chromosomes be studied but the individual genes that get corrupted can now be examined in many instances, and knowledge of the ways they can be cut and re-spliced with new bits of DNA to make new rogue genes is growing rapidly. Highly sensitive probes for the commoner rogue genes are available and now form an integral part of the work-up for any new case of leukaemia. *Cytogenetics* is the study of abnormal chromosomes and *molecular genetics* is the study of rogue genes.

Useful information can also be obtained simply by measuring the amount of DNA in the leukaemic cells. The amount of DNA in a cell is referred to as its state of *ploidy*. Normal cells are *diploid* which means they have a pair of each of the 23 chromosomes. Ova and sperm (see Chapter 2) are *haploid* which means they have only one of each of the 23 chromosomes. Cancer cells might be *hyperdiploid* (*hyper* = excess) where the number of chromosomes exceeds 46—there might be three of one chromosome or more, for example. The converse is seen where cells are *hypodiploid* (*hypo* = lack of) and contain fewer than 46 chromosomes.

So different subtypes of leukaemia are recognized by their profile which includes their clinical, morphological, immunophenotypic, and genetic features. The following chapters will describe the different leukaemias in more detail, how they are treated, and what happens to children who get them.

# 6
# Lymphoblastic leukaemia (ALL): the nature of the beast

Of all childhood leukaemias, most (80 per cent) are related to lymphocytes rather than granulocytes and are grouped together under the broad title of *lymphoblastic leukaemia*, or ALL for short. The 'A' is for acute but the word is superfluous because 'blastic' implies the same thing.

ALL is in fact a group of different diseases, the complexity of which is still being unravelled, and we have now reached the point where not all are treated the same. Using the techniques described in Chapter 5, for practical purposes ALL is presently divided into four categories based on *immunophenotype*. These are:

1. T ALL (where the cells have some of the characteristics of T lymphocytes);

2. B ALL (where the cells have the features of more mature B lymphocytes);

3. B precursor ALL (where the cells show the features of B lymphocytes arrested at an earlier stage in their development);

4. Early B precursor ALL (where the cells are showing the earliest possible signs of becoming B lymphocytes).

The four types thus defined have different symptoms and signs, the leukaemic cells may look different, and have different chromosome abnormalities. Most importantly, they have different responses to treatment and some are more curable than others.

The features that relate to response to therapy are described in detail in Chapter 7 and the clinical differences are outlined below in the section 'How ALL declares itself—the symptoms and signs'. The approximate proportion of each of the types is shown in Figure 2.

## Who gets ALL?

The chance of a child developing ALL is not equal throughout the years of childhood. There is a striking peak between the ages of 2 and

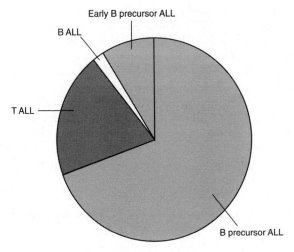

**Figure 2.** Proportions of different types of ALL occurring in children.

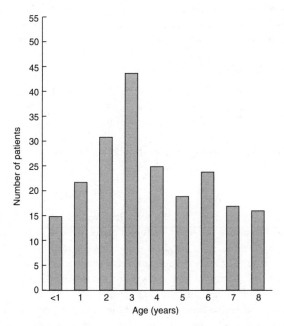

**Figure 3.** Age at diagnosis of 260 children with ALL from one region of the United Kingdom.

6 years as seen in Figure 3. The peak becomes more obvious if only the commonest type of B precursor ALL is considered, which means that very young infants and older children are relatively less likely to develop that subtype.

There is also an imbalance between the sexes with a slight but consistent excess of boys. They comprise about 55–60 per cent of all cases. This is true for all types of ALL, but is particularly striking in T ALL where boys account for around 80 per cent. Very young babies get ALL relatively rarely and the type they do get is often the early B precursor variety. ALL is, of course, not confined to childhood and occurs at all ages, but the commonest type of B precursor ALL is rare beyond the middle teens.

# How ALL declares itself—the symptoms and signs

The clinical features of ALL vary from type to type. Some symptoms and signs are common to all varieties, some are specific to one or another. The best way to recount the course of the disease is to break it down into the four types referred to above and to describe the typical features of each, noting where these are the same and where they differ.

## B precursor ALL

The commonest form of B precursor ALL (sometimes referred to as 'common' ALL) is an insidious disease that slowly develops over a long period of time, and it is only in the later stages that affected children become really ill. It affects principally children between 2 and 6 years of age, though can arise in those older and younger. There are a number of ways it can present itself.

### How it comes to light

'Common' B precursor ALL frequently causes a profound drop in haemoglobin before the white cells and platelets become low enough to cause problems. Such children may not be unwell, but are strikingly pale and the family doctor, suspecting anaemia (but not usually leukaemia), is prompted to carry out a blood count. From that the diagnosis becomes obvious or strongly suspected.

The gradual realization that 'something is wrong' is an equally frequent story. One of repeated visits to the family doctor, sometimes over many months, with non-specific problems of listlessness, pallor, loss of appetite, lack of energy, and repeated infections such as coughs, colds, and tonsillitis. Since such a story is very common among children who do *not* have leukaemia, and since leukaemia is so rare, it is not surprising that family doctors do not immediately leap to the diagnosis as their first conclusion.

As the disease progresses, bone marrow failure advances and, as well as the haemoglobin tumbling, the platelet count falls, and the neutrophils begin to disappear. Pallor becomes more pronounced and bruises may appear. Enlargement of the lymph nodes in the neck may be felt (though this is a common feature of innocent infections like tonsillitis and not in any way exclusive to ALL), and the patient's state of health continues to deteriorate.

Anaemia, though usually present to some degree, may go unnoticed before the platelet count collapses and the picture of a bleeding disorder appears. Children may occasionally present covered in bruises with nose and gum bleeding, but otherwise not particularly unwell.

It is unusual for children with 'common' ALL to be very ill or *in extremis* due to infection at the time the disease is first discovered. This is because the neutrophil count is the last thing to go as the disease progresses, and it is usually diagnosed before that stage is reached.

It is the event that provokes a blood count that dictates how leukaemia is discovered, for once that simple step has been taken, the diagnosis is usually obvious or strongly suspected. Occasionally it is done at an earlier stage than that of advanced bone marrow failure. One reason is bone pain. ALL, particularly 'common' ALL, sometimes causes aches and pains, particularly in the legs, hips, and back. The precise reason is not clear, but the source of the pain is the bones. When a child presents with this problem, perhaps associated with a limp or a reluctance to walk, it is common for referral to be made to specialists with an interest in rheumatic diseases or bone surgery.

X-ray examination may give the game away, as there are (fairly subtle) abnormalities to see in the growing bones of most children with ALL—fine translucent bands around the growing ends. But these can be missed if not specifically looked for. Sometimes the changes are more gross, and there can be quite extensive damage to the bones of (usually) the spine. This is found in children with stiff painful backs who present with a strikingly abnormal gait.

Apart from its effect on bones, which is perhaps how 5–10 per cent of children present, it is very unusual for 'common' ALL to come to light because of its effect on parts or systems of the body other than the bone marrow. Although other tissues may be infiltrated with leukaemic blast cells, this rarely produces symptoms.

Occasionally children with what eventually develops into 'common' ALL present with pallor and bone marrow failure as described above, not particularly unwell, but with a bone marrow empty of cells (normal or abnormal) creating the impression that they have aplastic anaemia (see Chapter 4). Sometime later (they may or may not partially recover in the meantime without treatment), the more typical picture evolves.

## Laboratory and clinical features at the outset

Children with 'common' ALL are usually pale, sometimes bruised, and may have enlarged lymph nodes in the neck, armpits, and groin that can be felt as rubbery little lumps varying in size from a pea to a broad bean. It may also be possible to feel their spleens (an indication of excessive size as normally spleens are tucked under the ribs on the left-hand side and cannot be felt), but otherwise there is usually little else remarkable to find.

Their blood counts are always abnormal. Anaemia is present in 99 per cent, and there is usually a neutropenia and thrombocytopenia. Leukaemic lymphoblasts can usually be found in the circulation but not always. When not, the diagnosis may not be immediately obvious and the picture may resemble aplastic anaemia. The total number of white cells (normal and abnormal) can be low, normal, or high. The normal range for white cells is $3–10 \times 10^9$ per litre of blood, and it is unusual for children with 'common' ALL to present with a count over 50.

The bone marrow is usually packed with lymphoblasts. The marrow may be difficult to suck out because 'common' ALL has a tendency to produce a matrix of tough scar-like tissue around itself. Occasionally it can be so stubborn in this respect that a marrow aspirate cannot be obtained and the diagnosis then rests on the trephine sample (see Chapter 4).

The pattern of immunological markers shows positivity for immature B cells but no features of more mature T or B cell characteristics. Genetic studies frequently show *hyperdiploidy*, where the leukaemic cells have extra chromosomes giving a total of 50 or more per cell.

Another large subgroup shows a small amount of material from chromosome number 12 transposed on to chromosome 21. This creates new genes that influence the growth pattern of the leukaemia. There are other genetic abnormalities in the remaining minority who have neither hyperdiploidy nor a 12;21 translocation; some are apparently random, others are seen regularly. The improvements in laboratory techniques means that more detailed knowledge about the range of genetic abnormalities seen is expanding quickly.

Around one child in 100 with 'common' B precursor ALL will have leukaemic cells (usually small numbers) in their spinal fluid, indicating infiltration of the central nervous system (CNS). The CNS includes the brain and spinal cord, is bathed in spinal fluid, and is well protected from the external environment. How the cells get in there is not known, but their presence is important as they can survive in peace and quiet, in an effective 'sanctuary', unless special steps are taken to deal with them.

## T ALL

T cell ALL presents a rather different picture from the common form of B precursor disease. It is much more frequent in boys—so much so that it was initially thought to be restricted to males. It also typically occurs at an older age—late childhood and early adolescence.

### How it comes to light

Unlike the immature B lymphocyte leukaemias, T ALL probably does not often *originate* in the bone marrow, but colonizes it as a secondary site at a later stage in its development. For that reason there is often much more evidence of leukaemic cells outside the confines of the marrow—blood blast cell counts are higher, lymph nodes are bigger, and spleens are more enlarged. There is a greater chance of finding blast cells in the CNS than in B precursor ALL. Also, perhaps because the marrow is not the primary seat of the disease, T ALL produces less bone marrow failure, so it is possible to have the cancer well advanced without bruising, bleeding, infection, or profound anaemia.

Cancers involving lymphocytes that replace lymph nodes, infiltrate spleens, livers, and other organs but that do not infiltrate the bone marrow to any great degree are not referred to as leukaemias but *lymphomas*. In children such cancers are very closely related to

ALL, and to call a T cell tumour lymphoma as opposed to leukaemia is a subtle distinction. Both are treated the same and probably represent small differences in the degree of maturity of the malignant cells.

For these reasons T ALL not infrequently presents as swelling in the neck. If that goes unnoticed or unrecognized, the disease will progress to a stage where bone marrow failure evolves and the triad of bruising, pallor, and infection emerge.

Occasionally the disease can present in a more dramatic way. Because T cells normally mature in the thymus gland, that organ is frequently enlarged in T ALL. It can be seen as an obvious shadow between the lungs on chest X-ray. The space between the lungs is known as the *mediastinum* and contains the heart, some big blood vessels, and the main windpipe, as well as the thymus and some lymph nodes around the roots of the lungs. The organs are tightly packed and there is very little room for expansion. X-ray visible enlargement of the nodes and/or thymus in ALL is referred to as a *mediastinal mass*. If such a mass is big enough it can obstruct the blood flow from the main vein of the body to the heart and the air supply to the lungs. For this reason T ALL is particularly liable to present as an emergency where the child will have engorged veins in the neck and noisy breathing due to partial blockage of the windpipe. Urgent treatment is needed. Occasionally a mediastinal mass is seen in other types of ALL.

## Laboratory and clinical features at the outset

Apart from the greater tendency to form lumps and bumps and to infiltrate the CNS and mediastinum, T ALL tends to present with a very high white blood cell count with large numbers of circulating blast cells. The count can be increased up to 50-fold or more.

Such high counts can occasionally affect the viscosity (stickiness) of the blood and alter its flow characteristics so that it sludges to a standstill in tiny blood vessels and fails to allow red cells carrying oxygen to reach the sensitive parts of the brain. The result of this can be varied, from a little mental dulling and deafness, through convulsions, to coma. Very occasionally the condition is fatal. It is called *leucostasis* (*leuco* = white cell, *stasis* = stoppage). The problem is more common in AML than in ALL.

T ALL is, by definition, positive for one or more immunological markers for T lymphocytes. The blast cells look similar to those from B precursor disease. Chromosome studies sometimes show abnormalities, some of which are only found in T ALL. Hyperdiploidy is not seen, nor the 12;21 translocation.

## B ALL

B ALL is very rare (1–2 per cent of all cases) and different from other types of ALL. Like T cell disease, it is in reality as much of a lymphoma as a leukaemia, but is also a highly malignant and aggressive tumour that is rapidly fatal if left untreated.

### How it comes to light

B ALL can present in a variety of ways, but the children are usually ill and have pains in the abdomen. The lymph nodes and lymphatic tissue in the intestines are a major seat for the disease, and afflicted children often have large masses of tumour that can easily be felt.

If extensive bone marrow involvement is present (which may or may not be the case—rather like T ALL), then failure supervenes fairly rapidly and bruising, pallor, and infection follow. The disease has a predilection for the CNS, so there is a relatively high chance of finding blast cells in the spinal fluid.

### Laboratory and clinical features at the outset

The blast cells of B ALL have a characteristic and striking appearance under the microscope. They also show the immunological characteristics of mature B lymphocytes and contain the building blocks for antibodies. They invariably have a peculiar and specific chromosome abnormality involving chromosomes numbers 8 and 14 where material has been swapped from one to the other, so have a genetic hallmark. One of the corrupted genes is that responsible for making parts of antibodies.

## Early B precursor ALL

This is much less clearly defined than the three types of ALL described above. It affects children of all ages, and is the type of ALL more frequently seen in adults.

There is one recognizable and important subgroup of early B precursor ALL that occurs in very young infants, usually less than 2 years old and often less than 1. The disorder is characterized by very high white blood cell counts, but without much lumpy disease as seen in T or B ALL. There is a very high rate of infiltration of the CNS as the disease progresses, and the hallmark of the syndrome is a chromosome abnormality involving numbers 4 and 11. There is a gene on chromosome 11 that is frequently corrupted in many different types of leukaemia. For this reason it is called the *mixed lineage leukaemia* or *mll* gene.

Early B precursor ALLs do not show the immunophenotype of B cells, but usually have some other CDs or features that allow them to be recognized as very immature B cells and thus a form of ALL. Occasionally they can be so poorly differentiated that there is doubt whether they are ALL or a featureless type of AML, but fewer and fewer leukaemias fall into that category as techniques for their recognition have become more sophisticated.

Once ALL has been diagnosed and classified as one of the above categories, therapy can begin. Before treatment became available the average time from diagnosis to death for such children was 3 months. Nowadays most survive the ordeal. Exactly how this has been achieved is explained in the next chapter.

# 7
# Lymphoblastic leukaemia: (ALL) the evolution of treatment and clinical trials

Childhood ALL has a unique place in the history of the struggle against cancer because it was the first malignant disease to show the value of drug treatment (chemotherapy) and the first to be cured by this means. The story starts in 1948 when doctors from the Harvard Medical School in Boston treated 16 terminally ill children with a new drug called *aminopterin*. Ten showed a good response and in some the disease disappeared completely, but this was only temporary and none were cured. Aminopterin was rather toxic, but a closely related compound, *methotrexate*, was developed soon after and remains an important component of treatment today.

During the 1950s and 1960s other drugs were found that were effective in treating ALL, including *6-mercaptopurine*, *6-thioguanine*, *steroids*, *vincristine*, *cyclophosphamide*, *cytarabine*, *asparaginase*, and the anthracyclines *daunorubicin* and *adriamycin*. These, plus the podophyllins *etoposide* and *tenoposide* developed in the 1970s, make up the arsenal of compounds used to treat ALL today. They are described in more detail below.

After aminopterin the next major advance was not a new drug, however. It was the discovery that giving more than one drug at once had an additive effect on the disease without additional harm to the patient. In the early 1960s this led to compound treatment programmes with strange acronyms like VAMP (vincristine, aminopterin, mercaptopurine and prednisone). Using repeated pulses of schedules of this type, long remissions were achieved in many children, but in most the disease eventually recurred and gradually became unresponsive to further treatment. Also, in children who survived long enough, a common problem that emerged was the appearance of leukaemic cells in the fluid surrounding the brain and the spinal cord (cerebro-spinal fluid (CSF) within the central nervous system (CNS)). This occurred because the drugs given by mouth or injected into the bloodstream did not penetrate the CNS, as the body has a very efficient 'blood:brain barrier'. Furthermore, once CNS leukaemia was established, it was very difficult to get rid of and usually led to the disease spreading once again to the bone marrow.

To tackle this problem, and to make temporary remissions more permanent, the most important milestone was the strategy developed in the 1960s at St Jude's Hospital in Memphis called 'total therapy'. This was the first attempt to eradicate the disease once and for all in a (for the time) daring schedule that included multi-drug treatment stretching over 2–3 years and early radiation therapy to the brain and spinal cord.

'Total therapy' had four components. First, the disease was made to remit with the least toxic treatment possible (*remission induction*). At the end of this phase the child would regain normal health and bone marrow function. The second phase was more aggressive with higher doses of drugs injected daily for a week to hit the disease as hard as possible (*remission consolidation*). The third phase was radiation therapy to the brain and spinal cord to treat cells in the CSF (*CNS directed therapy*), and the final phase, lasting up to 3 years, consisted of daily oral chemotherapy (*remission maintenance* or *continuing therapy*).

The St Jude's team reported their early results for this approach in 1971 and used the word 'cure' for the first time. By then eight of the first 37 children treated in this way had reached the fifth anniversary of their diagnosis without signs of disease recurrence despite having had no treatment for over 2 years. The word 'cure' has to be used with caution, however, since it subsequently became apparent that a few children relapsed with return of disease at a later stage than this. But most of the early survivors are still alive and well and nowadays there is no doubt that, for all practical purposes, children who get to the fourth anniversary of the completion of treatment and who are in their first remission can cautiously assume the disease has gone for ever.

The 'total therapy' philosophy and the same four phases of treatment survive to the present day, though many changes have been made. The drug schedules and combinations have been altered, newer drugs have been introduced, and radiation treatment has been largely abandoned in favour of other methods of treating the CNS in all but a few patients. Progress has been such that the point has now been reached where it can be claimed that most children with ALL can be cured.

Most, but not all. The majority of those who fail will do so because they have an intrinsically resistant type of disease. A minority will fail because, for one reason or another, the drugs do not work properly. Many factors can thus affect the outcome of treatment, some of which are evident at the outset. These *prognostic* factors (*prognosis* means foretelling the course of a disease) can therefore be used to identify children at high risk of treatment failure and to select them for alternative strategies. It should be clearly understood, though, that in the end treatment is the only prognostic factor, because on the one hand without it ALL is 100 per cent fatal and on the other if we had a perfect therapy everyone would be cured.

So prognostic factors only reliably relate to one treatment schedule. Having said that, some are so powerful that they emerge as important in most schedules that have been tried so far. They are discussed in more detail later. Before that it is important to consider the drugs used in more detail, to understand the rationale and nature of clinical trials, and to appreciate how modern treatment protocols are constructed.

# Drugs currently used in childhood ALL

Anti-cancer drugs work in various ways to stop cells dividing and to kill them by inducing them to commit suicide in the process of *apoptosis* (see Chapter 2). Because they kill cells they are collectively called *cytotoxic* (*cyto* = cell).

*Prednisolone* and *dexamethasone* are both steroid-based compounds. Not the body-building variety used by athletes, but with the function of suppressing inflammation (also used in diseases like arthritis to ease joint pain) and also with the capacity to destroy lymphoblasts in ways that are not properly understood. They are not damaging to normal cells in the same way as other drugs used, but they can induce a short remission in ALL even if given on their own. Their immediate side-effects include insomnia, increased appetite, mood changes, reversible muscle weakness and, occasionally, temporary diabetes, which recovers on stopping the drug.

*Methotrexate* is the modern derivative of aminopterin, and interferes with the formation of DNA in dividing cells. It is a relatively safe substance and can be injected into muscles or the spinal fluid, or taken by mouth without causing damage. It is removed by the kidneys and comes out in the urine. Large doses suppress normal bone marrow production causing neutropenia and thrombocytopenia. It is currently fashionable to inject very high doses into the blood and then give an antidote 24 hours later to 'rescue' normal marrow while (hopefully) inflicting irreversible damage on leukaemic cells. High doses also penetrate into the body's chemical sanctuaries including the brain and spinal cord.

*Vincristine* is a powerful drug obtained from the periwinkle *Vinca rosea*. It stops cells dividing during the actual process of the chromosomes splitting apart. It is a toxic substance and has to be injected directly into the bloodstream where it is rapidly diluted. If it is allowed to leak out of the vein during injection, it causes a nasty 'burn' in the skin. It should never be given by any route other than into a vein. There have been one or two tragic accidents where it has been given into the spinal fluid by mistake instead of methotrexate. Most children to whom this happens become totally paralysed and die. The drug causes slight weakness of (chiefly) the legs in some patients even if given correctly, and constipation due to partial bowel paralysis can also be a problem. Apart from its effect on nerves and muscles, it is well tolerated and does not cause low blood counts on its own. Some patients may temporarily lose their hair while receiving the drug at weekly intervals.

*6-Mercaptopurine* is a non-toxic compound that is usually taken by mouth. It has to be broken down in the body to become cytotoxic. Its active chemicals are produced inside cells and then prevent the formation of DNA, thus interfering with cell division. It has few side-effects other than low blood counts. There is a closely related compound called *6-thioguanine* which is also used and which is broadly similar in how it is given, its action, and side-effects.

*L-asparaginase* is different from other anti-cancer drugs in that, like steroids, it does not directly prevent cells from dividing so is not a cytotoxic drug in the conventional sense. Leukaemic lymphoblasts, to some extent, differ in their internal chemical make-up from normal cells, and asparaginase exploits those differences by removing a specific essential chemical which normal cells can replace but which leukaemic cells cannot. Thus deprived, the leukaemic cells die. The drug is an enzyme made in a cultured micro-organism (a bacterium), so it is more likely to provoke an allergic response than a synthetic laboratory-made compound. It also disturbs the body chemistry and occasionally causes problems with abnormal blood clotting, temporary diabetes, and inflammation of the brain causing seizures. The best scheduling and dosing of the drug are currently a matter of debate.

*Daunorubicin* and *adriamycin* are both drugs from the *anthracycline* family. They are powerful anti-leukaemic agents but are also very unpleasant substances. They cause severe burning and blistering if their injection into a vein leaks into the surrounding skin. They kill cells indiscriminately, and so depress bone marrow production and cause low blood counts. They also have the dangerous property of damaging the heart muscle, so the amount any one patient can have is limited. Heart damage may not be apparent at the time, and in children who have received too much can crop up years after treatment has finished, manifesting itself as heart failure. Research is currently being carried out to try to prevent this serious side-effect. The anthracyclines can produce nausea and vomiting for about 24 hours after an injection. They also cause temporary hair loss.

*Cyclophosphamide* is a distant relative of the sulphur mustard gas used during the First World War. (Nitrogen mustard, a closer relative, was the first chemical compound seen to have an effect on human cancer growth in the 1940s.) Like 6-mercaptopurine, it has to be activated within cells before it becomes cytotoxic, so is not unpleasant to handle. It can be taken by mouth or injected. It damages all cells, so causes bone marrow failure as a major side-effect. A peculiar problem with the drug is caused by a breakdown product that is discharged through the kidneys. The chemical involved causes inflammation of the bladder, pain on passing water, and blood in the urine. The problem is not seen with small infrequent doses, and can be prevented by another drug as an antidote, but, once established, can continue long after the drug is withdrawn. Cyclophosphamide also produces nausea and vomiting for 24–48 hours after a large dose, and temporary hair loss is usual. It is used in consolidation and maintenance therapy reinforcement blocks. Very large doses are used to prepare patients for bone marrow transplants (see Chapter 13).

*Etoposide* is derived from a compound found in the roots of the May Apple. As cytotoxic drugs go, it could be described as moderately unpleasant in that it is mildly irritant to skin if a vein injection site leaks, but it can also be taken by mouth. It kills normal as well as leukaemic cells (in ways that are incompletely understood), so causes cytopenias. It also causes hair loss (if other drugs have not already done so), but only produces nausea if high doses are injected. Oral treatment is usually well tolerated by out-patients.

*Cytarabine* (*cytosine arabinoside*) plays a larger role in AML than ALL (see Chapter 11), but is also used in most current ALL protocols to a varying degree. It inhibits DNA formation. At the conventional doses used for ALL therapy (high-dose therapy is used for AML), it has few unpleasant side-effects. It causes low blood counts, and occasional patients suffer nausea, fever, or skin rashes. The substance itself is not dangerous, and it can be given into the skin or spinal fluid as well as injected into veins.

Occasionally other cytotoxic drugs are used for ALL, but seldom for what might be called conventional 'front line' therapy. Antibiotics are used both to treat and prevent infection, and are considered in more detail in Chapter 12.

# Clinical trials: design and analysis

The progress from 100 per cent mortality to an odds-on chance of cure for ALL in the last 50 years (and the improved outlook for children with AML which will be covered in a later chapter) is entirely the result of experimental therapies and, latterly, carefully constructed clinical trials. In 1948 the original use of aminopterin in terminally ill children must have required extraordinary courage on the part of the children, the parents, and the doctors concerned. It almost certainly provoked criticism at the time for meddling with fatal diseases and prolonging a painful situation.

The ethics of experimental therapies and clinical trials have never been easy, particularly in children and in the context of a potentially fatal disease with all its attendant emotional difficulties. Nevertheless it is only by pursuing such adventures that progress can be made. The present day organization of clinical trials in childhood leukaemia has reached a level of sophistication and international collaboration that is unparalleled in cancer treatment, an impressive achievement that has been a process of evolution over several decades.

As anti-cancer drugs gradually became widely available in the 1950s it became standard practice to treat children with ALL rather than simply comfort them as they died, but there was little co-ordination. At first doctors in different hospitals gave what they thought best. In many countries the larger research hospitals (like St Jude's) pursued more structured trials of new drugs and drug combinations and some children were referred there for treatment but in a rather haphazard manner.

Gradually larger collaborative groups of interested doctors got together and designed clinical trials that allowed experience to be pooled and the answer to treatment-related questions to be gained more quickly. Mostly they were national groups and such organizations currently exist in all western European countries, the United States, Canada, Australia, and Japan. Their organization of clinical trials has proved very successful. For example, in the 1960s in the United Kingdom perhaps only 50 per cent of the children with ALL were treated in national trials. The figure today is approaching 100 per cent and the high standard of care offered by the 22 UK hospitals with specialist leukaemia units is very similar, all being involved in the same trials at the same time.

Now there is a growing trend towards collaborating on an international basis to design and conduct trials. The drive to do this is because very large numbers of patients are needed to get reliable answers to important questions about treatment, and the best way to do this is with large *randomized controlled trials*.

## Randomized controlled trials

The randomized controlled trial is a very powerful tool to discover which of two treatments is best. The principle is simple. A group of patients with the same disease are randomly allocated to one of two treatments. One treatment (A) will be the 'standard' approach and one (B) the new one under scrutiny. Patients on arms A and B are then compared for side-effects and outcome. 'Outcome' in terms of leukaemia is usually the proportion remaining disease free and in their first remission several years after diagnosis (see statistical analysis, below). For a consecutive series of trials the best arm of the first trial (say treatment B) is then compared with a new treatment (C) and so on. In complicated treatment schedules like those used to treat ALL, it is possible to compare more than two components of the programme and there may be two or more randomizations for each patient. In the current UK trial, for example, two different steroid types are being compared (dexamethasone and prednisolone), and two different drugs used in maintenance (6-mercaptopurine and 6-thioguanine). Children can therefore be allocated to either steroid or either maintenance drug, giving rise to four different combinations, but they can be studied as just two groups when comparing the results for either the steroid or the maintenance drug.

The trials are controlled because in any experiment it is important to have a known baseline (treatment A in the above example) which represents the current situation. It is not reliable simply to compare the results of a new leukaemia treatment given in 1995–8 with the old treatment given in 1992–5 (so-called historical control). This is because other things may have changed such as the quality of supportive treatment (new antibiotics, different blood transfusion policy, better X-ray facilities) which can also affect outcome. The two treatments have to be compared simultaneously.

Also important is the inclusion of all eligible children. If children are not entered into trials because (say) their parents or doctors feel they are not well enough, the eventual results may be over-optimistic because the most vulnerable patients would not be represented. This would be an example of *bias* in clinical trials.

All these points become more important as we are looking for smaller improvements in treatment outcome. For the original 16 children given aminopterin it did not matter that it was not a randomized controlled trial. For the first 37 given total therapy at St Jude's the same applies. Now, however, when we are looking for differences of 10 per cent or less in disease-free survival, the situation is very different and rigorously designed clinical trials are the only way confident progress can be made.

## Understanding statistical analysis

Statisticians play a major role in trial design and the decision about how long a given trial should continue. They can calculate how many patients will be needed to detect a defined level of difference (say a 10 per cent improvement for arm A over arm B) with a reasonable degree of confidence.

Apart from the large numbers of patients needed in most trials, another problem with clinical trials is the length of time it takes to get an answer to a therapeutic question. Say, for instance, that arm A produces a real 14 per cent advantage in long-term survival for children with ALL over arm B if the children are compared at 5 years from diagnosis. This means that the complete picture will not be available until 5 years after the last child enters the trial. The difference may only become apparent at 5 years, and there may be no such difference at (say) 3 years. Some differences may take even longer to emerge. Statisticians can help with this by performing an *actuarial* analysis of outcome. (An *actuary* is someone who works for a life insurance company and calculates the probability of mortality at various ages for potential customers and decides on the premiums they should pay.)

Actuarial analysis of survival at a defined time point uses all the available information to make a statistical best guess at what the true figure will be even if all the individuals contributing to the calculation have not reached the time point concerned. For example, take 100 children with ALL on a given treatment and assume you wish to calculate their actuarial 5-year survival. The first child may start treatment 2 years before the last one, as they will not all be diagnosed on the same day. After 2 years, some patients will have been followed for 24 months, some for only a few days.

By the time 5 years has been reached by the front markers, the most recent entries will be 3 years down the road. Some will have fallen by the wayside at various stages along the way. The 3-year survival figure will be absolute and known. Looking at the pattern of death between 3 and 5 years for those unlucky enough to perish in that period it will be possible to calculate an estimated proportion of the whole group that is likely to reach 5 years unscathed. The calculated figure will be more likely to be right the larger the numbers of patients and the longer they have been followed. Such actuarial analysis, and the comparison of observed to expected events arising in patients in trials, form the backbone of how questions are eventually answered.

Statistical analyses, if they show a difference, are said to be 'significant' or not depending on the probability of a difference arising by chance, and this is usually expressed as a '$p$' value ($p$ for probability). A '$p$' value of 0.05 or less means that the observed difference would arise by chance alone on less than five occasions in 100 (and a '$p$' value of 0.001 on less than one occasion in 1000).

Equally important, but less often quoted, are the confidence limits of an analysis. These are an estimate of the *size* of any observed difference and what its true value is likely to be. For example, in our 100 patients with a 14 per cent difference in survival, a statistical analysis that indicated the difference to be significant might have a '$p$' value of 0.02 (probability of chance result 2 in 100), but 95 per cent confidence limits could give values of 4 per cent to 24 per cent, suggesting that the true difference has a 95 per cent chance of lying between those two values and may not be as much as 14 per cent (or could be more). Small treatment differences, small numbers of patients, and short periods of time on treatment give rise to analyses that have borderline '$p$' values and wide confidence limits, common problems in childhood leukaemia trials.

## Other types of drug trials—new drugs under assessment

When pharmaceutical research laboratories discover new compounds that might or might not help patients with cancer, there comes a stage in the process when they have to be tried out on human volunteers. Depending on the stage of development, the volunteer trials are called *phase 1* and *phase 2* respectively. Phase 1 trials are designed to find what the side-effects are at varying doses and frequency of giving the drug. Once the best tolerated dose and frequency has been defined, phase 2 studies are designed to discover the effect (if any) the new drug has on various types of cancer. Such novel drugs are usually given on their own to patients who have some sort of measurable disease. The disease has to be measurable so that the response can be assessed.

Children with leukaemia who have blast cells in the blood can be used to see if the cells disappear when the drug is given. Phase 2 studies are therefore occasionally appropriate for children with end-stage resistant leukaemia and who are on palliative treatment. Phase 2 studies help in defining drugs that may be effective if given earlier in the course of disease in the context of a randomized trial (which is a phase 3 study).

The next chapter describes modern treatment protocol design and how ALL therapy is organized.

# 8
# Lymphoblastic leukaemia (ALL): current treatment schedules

It is impossible to describe every treatment protocol for childhood ALL currently in use throughout the world, but the fundamental principles of total therapy (remission induction, consolidation, CNS treatment, and maintenance) are common to all.

For treatment purposes it is usual to designate children as 'low', 'standard', or 'high risk'. This means that some children have features of their disease that categorize them as more or less likely to fail to respond to conventional treatment. This process of risk assessment is complicated because different doctors in different countries do it in subtly different ways. What is regarded as 'high risk' in Germany may not be in the United Kingdom, for example. This does not mean that the outcome of treatment is substantially different between countries—it isn't. Rather it reflects the fact that different experts look at the same problem from slightly different angles.

'High risk' is, of course, a relative term and based entirely on the observed outcome of previous treatments. In the UK at present it is defined in several ways. Some children have particular genetic abnormalities in the leukaemic cells—specific defective genes or groups of genes present in some cases but not in others and recognized from past experience to have sinister significance.

Others are recognized as disadvantaged by a combination of age, gender (boy or girl), and the circulating blood white cell count (WBC) at the time of diagnosis. These features relate to the likely outcome of treatment for virtually every trial protocol devised to date. An age/sex/WBC risk score was calculated by statisticians in Oxford from the outcome of a UK trial in 1985–90. This defines the 12 per cent of children who showed a long-term survival rate of less than 40 per cent. It is known as the Oxford hazard score and is depicted in Figure 4. What it tells us is that boys do less well than girls, progressively higher

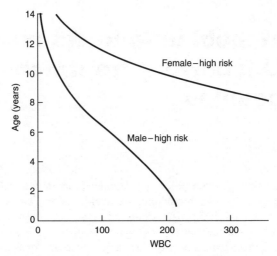

**Figure 4.** Thresholds that define high risk children with ALL (less than 40 per cent chance of long survival) based on age, gender, and diagnostic white count (WBC). This shows that an 8-year-old boy with a WBC of 200 × 10⁹/litre would thus be high risk whereas a girl of the same age would not. This graph is based on the Oxford hazard score. By permission of the author (Dr Sue Richards) and the British Journal of Haematology.

white counts relate to an increasing risk of treatment failure, and younger children respond better than adolescents.

There are other features that relate to outcome. These include initial disease responsiveness (rapid responders fare better than slow responders), great enlargement of the liver, spleen, and lymph nodes (the less the better), and the persistence of detectable traces of residual disease after several weeks or months of treatment. In many children, such *minimal residual disease* (MRD) can now be detected with great sensitivity where one leukaemic cell in a million normal cells can be identified. This is done by looking for traces of an abnormal genetic fingerprint of the disease defined at the time of diagnosis. The technology is still in its early stages, but has already reached the point where some trial designers are using it as a tool to put children into risk groups and so alter therapy.

Children regarded as high risk, however defined on any criteria, are usually given some alternative to the standard therapy. The protocol is usually similarly structured and given over a similar period of time as for standard risk, but is invariably more intensive. The words 'aggressive' or 'intensive' refer to chemotherapy that is given in higher doses or with more drugs being combined (or both), and which usually produces more prolonged and profound bone marrow suppression. Short-term side-effects (nausea, infections, and bleeding) are therefore more frequent and more hospital-based supportive treatment is needed. Despite more intensive schedules, high risk patients still fare less well than standard risk children, and the challenge they present is one of the most active areas of clinical research.

Also excluded from 'standard risk' trials are the 1–2 per cent of children with mature B cell ALL (see Chapter 6). These rare children do not respond well to conventional total therapy, but do much better with a short (6-month) schedule of aggressive multi-drug chemotherapy consisting of six or more pulses of combined drugs. They do not require a long period of maintenance treatment. The mature B cell variety is best regarded as a completely different disease from other types of ALL.

# The timetable of conventional treatment for ALL

What follows is a brief synopsis of the pattern of therapy currently employed for 'standard risk' patients which comprise 75–80 per cent of the total numbers of children with ALL. Readers should understand that there are many variations on the same theme in use throughout the world with alternative timings and design but which do not differ substantially in principle.

For 24 hours prior to beginning treatment, children are given a drug called *allopurinol*. This is given in anticipation of a large amount of cell breakdown products soon to be floating around the bloodstream and having to be dumped to the outside via the urine. Allopurinol helps the waste to stay dissolved and avoids it crystallizing out and blocking the delicate filtration beds in the kidneys. For the same reason large amounts of intravenous fluids are given to make sure the kidneys have a brisk flow through them established.

The first drugs to be given are usually vincristine and steroids, together with a dose of methotrexate into the spinal fluid. Vincristine is given as four injections at weekly intervals, and steroids as pills every day. Asparaginase is also given as a remission induction drug, usually as an injection into the leg skin or muscles, 9–12 times over the first 4 weeks. The fluid flush and allopurinol can be stopped after the first day or two. The marrow will usually be re-examined after 1 week to see if the disease is clearing rapidly or slowly. This may be important as an indicator of later outcome.

Remission (normal blood counts and normal marrow recovery) is usually achieved after 4 weeks. This does not mean that the disease has completely gone—it hasn't at that stage—it indicates simply that it has reduced in amount sufficiently to allow normal organ functions to resume and health to return.

At diagnosis there will be something like $10^{12}$ malignant cells in the body of a 7-year-old child with ALL. That is, 1000 billion cells weighing about a kilogram and occupying the equivalent space of something like a medium sized melon. Reducing that to one-thousandth of its original size would leave a single gram of disease smaller than an orange pip. That is what happens by the time remission is achieved, but there are still $10^9$ cells left—a billion—so there is much work to do before there can be any talk of cure.

The next phase is usually some form of consolidation treatment, more intensive or sustained chemotherapy designed to reduce the number of cells another 1000-fold. The drugs commonly used include daunorubicin, cytarabine, etoposide, and cyclophosphamide. Consolidation produces bone marrow failure during which blood counts will be low and supportive therapy in the form of blood or platelet transfusions or antibiotics will usually be needed. In anticipation of this most patients will have had a central venous catheter inserted during the first week or two of treatment to make supportive treatment easier (see Chapter 12).

Before or after consolidation comes therapy directed at the central nervous system (CNS). Lumbar punctures with direct injection of chemotherapy into the spinal fluid will have already been done at diagnosis and on several other occasions by this stage, but that is not regarded as sufficient. Further treatment may consist of a course of weekly lumbar punctures with or without two or three very high doses of intravenous methotrexate with rescue after 24 hours using the antidote folinic acid. The rationale of this is that very high blood concentrations of methotrexate allow the drug to penetrate into the CNS. Normally there is an effective blood:brain barrier to noxious chemicals as part of the body's defence mechanisms, but this unfortunately also protects the leukaemic cells that may have crept into this so-called 'sanctuary' site.

A few older children with high white counts (marking them at higher risk of CNS involvement) may receive radiation therapy to the brain. This treatment, though effective, is less widely applied than it was because of concerns over long-term side-effects as described in Chapter 16. It used to be used in all children.

Following the CNS phase, all children except those given radiation therapy continue to have occasional lumbar punctures throughout the rest of their treatment programme. Radiation recipients are spared because there is no evidence that extra methotrexate is beneficial and for them it may add to long-term toxicity.

After CNS directed therapy is complete, the maintenance phase of treatment begins, and usually consists of daily tablets of 6-mercaptopurine (started during the CNS phase), together with weekly tablets of methotrexate and monthly injections of vincristine coupled with 5-day pulses of steroid tablets. Further consolidation intensive blocks may be given later.

This prolonged daily therapy with oral drugs appears to be very important for the cure of the commoner types of childhood ALL. It is curious, because no other human cancer responds to this type of treatment and it flies in the face of experience with chemotherapy in other tumours. The original rationale of the designers of 'total therapy', who first mooted a long 'maintenance' phase of treatment, was to echo the experience of treating tuberculosis, where prolonged treatment with antibiotics is needed to cure the condition. But tuberculosis is an infection and ALL is a cancer, two fundamentally different disease processes. So the early treatment pioneers did the right thing for the wrong reason, and all attempts to curtail or dispense with this component of ALL treatment have led to a higher incidence of resistant disease and an increased number of relapses.

Maintenance treatment continues to 2 years (some schedules are for 3), during which time children have to attend clinics regularly to have the doses of their 6-mercaptopurine and methotrexate adjusted according to whether they have any cytopenias indicating a reduction in dose to be necessary.

At that stage treatment is stopped. The patient then enters what some call the 'observation phase' where regular clinic visits are maintained and a watch kept for signs of disease recurrence. The opportunity is also taken to monitor growth, development, and the evolution of any late side-effects. Initially patients may be seen at monthly intervals, but after a year or two the frequency of attendance will fall at a rate dependent on factors like travel distance and whether there are any active clinical problems.

# Immediate side-effects of treatment

Some of the immediate problems associated with ALL therapy are considered here. The long-term effects of treatment are mulled over later (Chapter 16) and details of supportive therapy (preventing and fighting infections, transfusing blood and blood components, nutritional support, and the sharing of care when children live a long distance from their treatment centre) are given in Chapter 12.

## Remission induction

Occasionally the response to early therapy can be dramatic and massive cell breakdown occurs at a rate that overwhelms the body's waste disposal system, despite a good fluid flush and allopurinol. The problem is called 'tumour lysis syndrome'. The kidneys fail, becoming clogged up with waste sludge, and temporary use of some artificial kidney system may be needed. Usually the kidneys recover quite quickly. Very occasionally there is such a dramatic and intolerable chemical upheaval in the body's internal environment that it proves fatal. Unfortunately there is little that can be done to make treatment more 'gentle' to overcome the hazard. Indeed, in a tiny number of ill children with well advanced disease the kidneys may already be struggling before treatment due to death of leukaemic cells in the process of their natural turnover.

Once the danger of too-rapid response is passed, remission induction is usually trouble free. Infection or bleeding at this stage is usually a complication of the disease rather than the treatment.

## Consolidation

The drugs used in most consolidation programmes will cause hair loss. They also cause short-term nausea and vomiting, but that can usually be controlled by other drugs to suppress this otherwise distressing side-effect. The main problem at this stage is the bone marrow production failure that follows any 'intensive' therapy. Very low neutrophil counts can persist for up to 3 weeks during which time serious infections can arise. Low platelet counts can cause troublesome bleeding.

## Treatment of the CNS

The side-effects of this phase of therapy depend, of course, on whether it consists just of spinal fluid methotrexate, whether additional high-dose intravenous methotrexate is also given, or whether radiation therapy is used instead. Spinal fluid methotrexate seldom causes symptoms though occasionally headaches and irritability are seen.

High-dose intravenous methotrexate is also without side-effects, provided the antidote rescue proceeds smoothly. Normal kidney function is essential to allow the excess methotrexate to escape from the body. If for some reason it doesn't, and if the antidote is withdrawn too early, the result is profound bone marrow failure with painful sores in the mouth, gullet, stomach, and intestines. For this reason the blood level of methotrexate is always carefully measured before the antidote is stopped.

Deep X-ray therapy to the brain causes little immediate trouble except for a few days' drowsiness some 6–8 weeks later. The degree of this so-called 'sleepy syndrome' is variable from patient to patient. Any hair that a child might have managed to retain falls out after the X-rays have finished, and complete baldness is invariable. The regrowth time is around 6 months.

## Maintenance

Apart from the disruptive effects of any additional blocks of 'intensive' treatment and their consequent bone marrow failure, infections, and bleeding, maintenance treatment is generally trouble free. Intercurrent infections arise from time to time, usually due to viruses. Most are trivial and get better on their own if treated with a little patience, but some, notably chickenpox and measles, are more of a worry. (See *Infection and lymphopenia* in Chapter 12.)

# The outcome of treatment and probability of long survival

Given the best currently available treatment over 75 per cent of children in the standard risk category will remain in apparently permanent remission and be cured of their disease. Even taking all risk categories together, the proportion achieving 10 years in first remission now exceeds 60 per cent (see Figure 5), and the survival curve is still rising gently.

But relapse is still all too common, frequently occurs unexpectedly, and the treatment of relapsed disease is far from satisfactory, as will become clear in the next chapter.

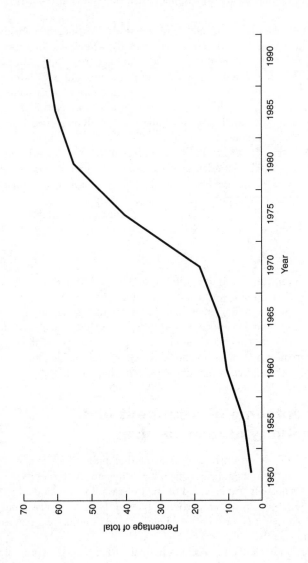

# 9
# Lymphoblastic leukaemia (ALL): relapse and its management

All but a very few children with ALL will respond to treatment to begin with. The blast cells will disappear from their blood and bone marrow over the first 2 or 3 weeks, and they will go into remission from their disease. As noted before, however, there is a world of difference between remission and cure. In remission, despite apparent normal health there may still be a billion malignant leukaemic cells lurking somewhere in the body. For cure, they all need to have vanished or to have lost their malignant potential—that is the capacity to grow outside the body's normal control.

When a remission becomes a cure can only be defined with confidence after the passage of time. There is no way of knowing exactly when the last blast cell has gone or whether the few remaining cells have lost their capacity to divide.

Relapse is defined as the reappearance of leukaemia in a patient previously in remission. It occurs for one of two reasons. Either the disease is intrinsically resistant to the treatment that has been given, or the treatment has not been given effectively. In other words, the drugs simply do not work or have not been given a proper chance to. Most relapses fall into the former group. Clear examples are seen in children whose disease recurs after only a brief remission of a few weeks or months. A few fall into the latter group. They include children who relapse later and who may have defaulted on taking their maintenance medication. This is a particular problem in undeveloped countries but also occasionally arises elsewhere.

Relapse is a devastating development at any stage, and the earlier it occurs the worse the outlook for the child concerned. The commonest way the disease reappears is to creep back into the bone marrow and cause unexplained low blood counts, or for blast cells to reappear in the blood. It can also reappear elsewhere in the body. It has a predilection for the central nervous system (CNS). In boys it also not uncommonly crops up in the testes, and rarely, it can singly involve other organs like the eye. These events are described in more detail below, but in short, relapse can arise in different ways, in different organs, and at different times, and exactly how, when, and where it appears influences how it is managed.

There is a small group of children, usually in 'high risk' groups (see Chapter 8), who fall by the wayside quite early on in the first 6–12 months, and they usually rapidly redevelop bone marrow infiltration and failure with low blood cell counts. The reappearance of disease at this early stage is a very sinister development following which successful 'salvage' treatment is very unlikely. Relapse while on therapy, though, is much less common than it used to be and most children who relapse do so after the end of treatment.

Currently, the risk of relapse after successfully completing treatment appears to be of the order of one in four to one in five. The risk is greatest in the first 2 years of therapy after which it diminishes gradually with the passage of time. After 4 years off treatment the risk becomes very small. At what point it becomes zero is impossible to say, as there are odd anecdotal reports of very late relapses after 10 years or more. These rare events raise the query whether the disease has truly relapsed or is a new leukaemia, but there is good evidence that such relapses *do* seem to be a recurrence of the original disease.

# Symptoms and signs of relapse at different sites

## Relapse in the bone marrow

Most frequently, ALL recurs by producing the same symptoms and signs as it did at the outset. Because patients are under closer medical scrutiny at the time of relapse, though, the problem tends to get picked up earlier and may be discovered by a perturbation in one of the routine blood counts. There may, alternatively, be a recurrence of original symptoms, like leg pains, fatigue, or something of which the child complains that may bring the problem to light. Either way, the blood will be abnormal and the suspicion can be confirmed by bone marrow examination.

## Relapse in the CNS

The brain and spinal cord are covered in a delicate layer of thin waterproof linings called *meninges*—a protective device vaguely similar to a tailored triple bag of fine polythene. The clear spinal fluid is found between the inner two membranes, and it is here that bacteria can invade to cause *meningitis*. Leukaemic cells can also grow in this carefully protected environment. Unless directly injected, drugs fail to penetrate the spinal fluid because of a chemical blood:brain barrier that exists to protect the CNS from toxic substances.

Central nervous system relapse usually declares itself in a way similar to mild meningitis—with headaches and early morning vomiting often without nausea. Occasionally it can be more insidious and present with an abnormally increased appetite, fatness, and sleepiness, though how it produces such an effect is not clear. Seizures (fits) are not common as an initial feature, probably because ALL does not usually directly invade the brain itself and damage it. The disease simply colonizes the meninges and eventually envelops or cloaks the whole of the outside of the brain and cord. Pressure changes can occur inside the skull and the flow of spinal fluid can become obstructed, and this can sometimes cause fits.

Isolated CNS relapse (i.e. not associated with marrow infiltration at the same time) currently arises in about 5–7 per cent of patients. It can occur at any stage after the beginning of treatment, though seldom arises more than 2 years off treatment. It is more likely to arise in children who had a very high white cell count at diagnosis—particularly very young infants. It is also more common in those with T ALL, irrespective of their initial white count.

## Relapse in the testis (testicle)

It has been well known for many years that boys with ALL can turn up at any stage with painless enlarged testes (one or both, often asymmetrical) as the first and sometimes the only sign of recurrent disease. The problem can arise at any stage, even some years after treatment has finished.

Why the testis is a particular target is not clear. There has been much 'harbour or harbinger' debate about whether the phenomenon is due to the fact that the testes are obvious to see and feel and testicular relapse indicates nothing more than organ infiltration outside the bone marrow that just happens to be more visible in boys, or whether the testis, like the CNS, is a true 'sanctuary' site where leukaemic blasts can lurk in safety protected from the drugs due to some unique 'blood:testis barrier'. Presently the sanctuary theory is less favoured. Whatever the cause, it is important that all boys have a careful physical examination at regular intervals during and for several years after their programme of treatment.

## Other sites of relapse

The eye is a rare site where ALL can show the first signs of its recurrence. The affected eye (usually one, but sometimes both) is often red and painful, with or without some loss of vision. Careful examination with the proper equipment can show leukaemic blast cells in front of the lens of the eye. Some consider this remote part of the body to be another 'sanctuary' for blast cells, but the problem is too unusual for there to be any clear indication one way or the other.

In girls, the ovary can become infiltrated, but because it is not visible or in a position where it can be felt, it seldom appears as a site of isolated relapse, though such cases have been seen. The enlarged organ, normally the size of a broad bean, has produced problems when the dimensions of a cricket ball are reached by causing an obstruction, pain, or a visible swelling.

Relapse can occur at more than one site at once, of course, and it is quite possible to have CNS leukaemia discovered concurrently with a marrow relapse. It is vitally important to have a good look round everywhere if there appears to be a simple isolated pocket of disease in one organ.

# The treatment of relapse

What can be done, and what the outlook is, depends more on the timing of the relapse than on the site. The later a relapse occurs the greater the chances are of being able to do something about it. Second and subsequent relapses are much more difficult, and require separate consideration.

Two principles are important to remember when planning any rescue treatment. First, there is no such thing as a 'slight' relapse. Either the disease has re-emerged or it has not. If it has, the second point to be clear about is that ALL is a whole body disease. Just because a patient has (say) an isolated testicular relapse does not mean that that is the only site of active disease, even if the bone marrow and spinal fluid (which should always be examined in such circumstances) are apparently clear. In other words relapse is an absolute state and to refer to an 'isolated' relapse means that the *symptoms* and *signs* are isolated, not the underlying disease.

It is hard to generalize about the treatment of relapse and plans should always be tailored to the individual. Wherever curative salvage is attempted it is important that questions are asked in clinical trials in just the same way as first time treatment (see Chapter 7) if any real progress is to be made.

## Treatment of bone marrow relapse while on treatment or within 3 months of its completion

Patients who relapse in the first year of treatment form a large proportion of those in the 'high risk' groups. Others are children with unexpectedly truly resistant disease. They should be vigorously treated with different drugs, doses, and schedules, and considered as candidates for some form of bone marrow transplant procedure (see Chapter 13). The exact schedule followed is less important than the principle. Most patients will remit again in such circumstances, but it is the maintenance of the second remission that is the difficult part.

Those not able to have a bone marrow transplant have a very high incidence of further relapse, and their second remission is seldom longer than the first. Those who receive a transplant have a higher risk of premature death from treatment-associated problems, and still have a depressingly high incidence of further relapse. Very few children who relapse early on treatment become long survivors whatever treatment is given, and they present one of the biggest challenges.

Children who relapse towards the end of the second year of treatment or shortly after its conclusion will still include a high proportion with truly resistant disease but will also consist of an increasing number who have received inadequate therapy for one reason or another. For that reason the results of treatment compared with those relapsing earlier will be slightly better. Second remissions will be longer, though based on present experience the likelihood is that nearly all will eventually relapse again.

## Treatment of bone marrow relapse occurring late after completion of treatment

The late relapse of ALL (over 2 years off treatment) suggests that the disease is not resistant to first line therapy, but that its eradication has been incomplete. Second remissions are easy to achieve in such circumstances, and can be maintained for long periods of time, but are still hard to turn into long-term cures. Whether a more aggressive programme of conventional chemotherapy or some form of marrow transplant offers the best treatment option is an area of current uncertainty.

Unlike the 'high risk' relapsers, patients in the long-off-therapy group have a lot to lose in terms of years of remission if a transplant goes wrong (see Chapter 13). On the other hand, if they are merely given a second programme of therapy exactly like the first, there is a near certainty of a second relapse, and, like the 'high risk' group, if that happens, the duration of the second remission is usually shorter than the first. For this reason there is every encouragement to be whole-hearted in the treatment of late relapsers. Using the most aggressive current schedules a substantial proportion may be salvaged, even without bone marrow transplantation.

## Treatment of CNS relapse

Isolated CNS leukaemia can usually be made to disappear and its symptoms to subside by one or two weekly injections of methotrexate into the spinal fluid. Long remissions can subsequently be achieved by giving deep X-ray treatment to the brain (if that has not been done already) and maintained by periodic injections of more methotrexate or 'triple' spinal fluid therapy with methotrexate, cytarabine, and steroids. The problem is indolent, however, and further CNS relapses are likely to occur albeit after some considerable time.

All this treatment, plus the leukaemia itself, is potentially damaging to the delicate structure and function of the brain and cord. Children with CNS disease who have had two or three recurrences, high doses of X-rays, and many injections of drugs into the spinal fluid often show some signs of damage by a tendency to fits and dulling of their mental processes. An unlucky few may develop more serious problems with progressive brain failure and severe mental handicap.

The end result of repeatedly relapsing CNS disease is usually an eventual bone marrow recurrence, poor control of that, and an inexorable slide into bone marrow failure leading to death. Very occasionally such children perish as a direct result of the CNS problem while the bone marrow is still uninvolved.

Whether children who have an isolated CNS relapse are best treated by bone marrow transplantation is not clear, but the option is worth considering.

## Treatment of testicular relapse

Isolated infiltration of the testis in boys with ALL usually occurs late, after therapy has been completed, and so is essentially a variant of long-off-treatment relapse.

Testicular relapse is not an indolent problem like CNS disease. It is probable that a higher proportion of boys with an isolated recurrence of this type can be salvaged (i.e. cured) than any other children with relapsed ALL, though success in this respect can only be achieved by a full programme of aggressive total body treatment. Whether it is always necessary to give radiation therapy to the testes is not entirely clear, though it is custom and practice to do so. Any boy receiving this will subsequently become sterile.

Testicular relapse occurring early during treatment does occasionally arise and is a totally different problem. It carries the same sinister outlook as any other recurrence at that stage and requires equally drastic measures.

## Treatment of relapse in the eye or elsewhere

The outlook for relapse in unusual isolated sites is essentially the same as for testicular disease. The principles of treatment are also the same and involve a programme of whole body therapy sufficiently different from the first to be an alternative together with some concentrated treatment, usually deep X-rays, to the affected part—the eyes, a particularly affected bone, or whatever. Such children are rare, and it is difficult to estimate the chances of long-term success on any grounds other than the length of time from the original diagnosis—the longer the better.

## Treatment of second or subsequent relapse

In normal circumstances, where the approach to primary treatment and that of first relapse has been adequate by current standards, the appearance of a further recurrence is a serious event that carries a very poor outlook in the short to medium term. For such unfortunate children treatment plans have to be carefully drawn up on an individual basis. They may be eligible for a marrow transplant in a third remission if they have not had one before. If not, they may be suitable for phase 1 or 2 trials of new drugs (see Chapter 7).

For the majority, however, and particularly for those children relapsing after a marrow transplant in their second remission, the outlook is grim. If experimental therapies fail or are not appropriate, then palliation becomes the aim of treatment. Here the ambition should be to maintain well-being and to keep children as well as possible and out of hospital as much as possible.

While further remission might be achieved, this should be attempted using treatment schedules that can be applied to children while out of hospital. Weekly injections of vincristine together with daily oral steroids will suffice in many instances. Third or subsequent remissions can then be maintained, often for surprisingly long periods of time, with home-based supplies of 6-mercaptopurine and methotrexate being controlled with fortnightly hospital visits just as in the first remission schedule. Admissions to hospital are reserved for actual illness. Even in the face of active persisting disease, good control for long periods of time can sometimes be achieved with oral drugs such as pulses of steroids and low-dose oral etoposide.

The management of ALL when the clear aim is palliation rather than cure can be described as the phase of pre-terminal care. This phase can last for months or, in some cases, years. If handled skilfully, it can shorten the final phase and make the transition to the last hurdle easier and more acceptable for the child and the whole family.

## Terminal care in relapsed ALL

When a child with ALL proves to have disease that no longer responds to any kind of treatment, when terminal marrow failure creeps in and the need for blood transfusions, platelets, and antibiotics escalates, the end is not far off. It is important that everyone recognizes the fact, and that plans are made, as at all other stages of treatment, for how to manage the inevitable event. The psychology of the situation is discussed in Chapter 15, but there are some practical aspects to be clear about.

Pre-terminal and terminal leukaemia is not often painful in the same way that other cancers can be, though children who feel wretched will frequently complain of pain because they cannot analyse their symptoms. Occasionally there can be genuine widespread bony aches and pains, but these often do not need the same doses of powerful pain killers that adults with lung or breast cancers frequently require.

While the pre-terminal phase may be very drawn-out, the last phase may be quite short and last only a matter of days or weeks.

Children with leukaemia may be reasonably well right up to the last 24 or 48 hours. As the disease advances, the threat to life comes from marrow failure, and in particular the twin risks of infection and bleeding. The terminal event is often a combination of the two, sometimes involving the lungs or brain. In that event it is usually fairly rapid unless inappropriate attempts at resuscitation and life-support in an intensive care unit are applied.

From being well, a child might develop some serious symptom (such as pain, shortness of breath, diarrhoea, vomiting, seizure, or altered consciousness). The next stage is also difficult to predict, but over some hours or days most children slide into a half-conscious dream-like state where they may be aware of who is around them but not what is happening. They may become restless in the last day or two of life, and if that happens, or if bone pain is troublesome, it is common practice to give the drug *morphine* or some close relative. This not only relieves pain but also creates a euphoric and detached state of mind and allows the child to remain comfortable. Gradually consciousness slips away, and breathing may become laboured before finally it stops.

If there is no defined terminal event like a bleed into the brain, patients will often become ill with a raised temperature, and will deteriorate over a few days, sliding into what is descriptively called '*progressive multisystem failure*'. One by one the vital body systems (liver, kidneys, lungs, brain) falter and fail and the same dream-like state described above is reached.

# 10

# Acute myeloid leukaemia (AML): the nature of the beast

The description in Chapter 1 is of one of the many ways acute myeloid leukaemia (AML) can present and emphasizes the way it often differs from the usually more insidious onset of ALL, though to distinguish the two types of acute leukaemia on the initial clinical picture can be difficult.

AML is a very mixed group of diseases—more so than ALL. *Myeloid* literally means 'marrow-like', and in this context simply means arising from developing blood cells in the marrow. Essentially, the term AML embraces all leukaemias that are related to blood cells *other than* lymphocytes—in other words those involving immature neutrophils, monocytes, and, occasionally, eosinophils and basophils. It also includes malignant growths of *megakaryocytes*, the platelet-producing cells, and, very rarely in children, of the developing red cells or *erythroblasts*. The latter condition is called *erythroleukaemia*, a perhaps rather illogical name that literally means red white blood.

AML is thus a generic term embracing all these disorders. To emphasize that it means 'all leukaemias other than ALL' it is sometimes referred to as ANLL—*acute non-lymphoblastic leukaemia*. There are specific subtypes that are usually given more precise names, like erythroleukaemia, above. Another example is *acute promyelocytic leukaemia*, where the cells are developed to the stage of *promyelocytes* (see Chapter 4). There is a type involving just monocytes sometimes called *acute monocytic leukaemia*. *Megakaryoblastic* leukaemia is usually referred to by that name, and a growth involving neutrophils and monocytes together is called *myelomonocytic* leukaemia.

## Who gets it?

AML in children is much less common than ALL. Between birth and 15 years of age the chances of developing some form of the disease are no more than one in 8000. There are less than 100 new cases in the whole of the UK each year, and AML collectively comprises only some

10–14 per cent of childhood leukaemia, though it may be commoner in some parts of the world than in others—in Africa and Japan, for example.

It does not have a well-defined peak age of risk like ALL, and the proportion of children who develop it is pretty constant up to the age of puberty. Beyond childhood, the incidence gradually rises with advancing years such that between 30 and 40 the risk is over four times as great, and rises sharply again over the age of 50. From the age of 20, in most countries, AML becomes more common than ALL. For this reason AML is often referred to as the 'adult' type of acute leukaemia.

## What causes it?

AML is known to be more common in children with some rare predisposing diseases such as Down syndrome, neurofibromatosis, Fanconi's anaemia, or Bloom's syndrome. Why is less clear. Also, occasionally, the problem arises as a result of previous anti-cancer drugs, or toxic chemicals when it is referred to as *secondary* AML—a special category considered separately below. Otherwise little is known about the cause or causes.

In parallel with the increasing incidence of AML in old age, there is an increasing frequency of aberrant growth patterns of elderly bone marrow cells unassociated with any illness but detectable with sophisticated laboratory investigations, and these patterns may provide a clue in the future. It is also perhaps relevant that the tempo of AML is more variable than that of ALL. More often it is the end result of a pre-existing blood disorder initially not frank acute leukaemia but slowly evolving into it over a period of months or years (*myelodysplastic syndromes*, see Chapter 14).

These features suggest that the disease is a result of some disruption in the orderly replication of bone marrow stem cells necessary for the continued uninterrupted supply of neutrophils, red cells, and platelets. But, outside the context of secondary leukaemia, exactly what that disruption is due to is not known, and claims that environmental radioactivity or any other pollutant might be responsible are entirely speculative at present.

## What types there are

AML is traditionally subdivided on the basis of the symptoms and signs and the appearance of the leukaemic blast cells under the microscope. The microscopically visible features of the blast cells have been categorized by a group of French, American, and British experts referred to as the FAB panel. There are eight different FAB types, given the codes FAB M (for myeloid) 0–7. Some of the distinctions are subtle, other types show more radical differences.

Whereas immunological cell typing (sorting cells by specially made anti-cell antibodies, see Chapter 5) has been of great value in the sub-categorization of ALL, in AML it has been perhaps of less help. This is because there are many more antibodies reacting with many more leukaemic cell features making the whole thing rather confusing. There are some subtypes where the technique is particularly helpful, however—types M0 and M7.

Chromosome studies, on the other hand, have been particularly valuable in AML. There are many chromosome abnormalities described that are associated either with myeloid leukaemias in general or with specific AML subtypes and some of these are import-ant in terms of predicting response to treatment.

So the categorization of AML is presently a combination of *mor-phology* (what the leukaemic cells look like with various stains under the microscope), *immunology* (what special antibodies react with in the leukaemic cells), and *genetics* (what chromosome or genetic abnormalities the leukaemic cells have). But whereas with ALL the dominant discriminant is *immunology*, with AML it is still traditional microscope *morphology* with the major consideration being what the cells look like, and the various disorders are referred to by their FAB type.

## M0 and M1 AML

The distinction between M0 and M1 AML is subtle and probably clinically unimportant. Both are highly malignant tumours of imma-ture neutrophils, with M0 cells showing less signs of maturity than M1, but not much. M0 cells are so featureless it can sometimes be hard to be certain that they are neutrophil related rather than repre-senting an atypical ALL, and that is why immunological cell typing can be particularly helpful in such circumstances. The two types combined account for some 20 per cent of AML cases in children.

Typical of most types of AML, M0/M1 disease usually presents with some evidence, often dramatic, of bone marrow failure with bleeding, anaemia, or infection, or some combination of these. It can arise at any age in childhood. The lymph nodes and spleen are seldom more than slightly enlarged, unlike ALL, though occasionally the tonsils may be big through associated infection. Like ALL, it can involve the spinal fluid, though does so much, much less commonly. Adults very rarely show spinal fluid involvement.

## M2 AML

The pedigree of M2 AML is more obvious with the leukaemic cells actually looking like very primitive neutrophils. Also it is in the M2 variant that the classic hallmark of the disease can be seen most frequently in the cytoplasm of the blast cells. These are Auer Rods. They are abnormal granules visible on high powered light microscopy and appear as fine red splinters inside the cells. They are named after the German pathologist who first described them and are only seen in leukaemia. They are therefore a very useful landmark in diagnosis. They are seen in other types of AML, notably M3 disease (see below), and in myelodysplastic syndromes. They are never seen in ALL.

M2 is the commonest subtype of AML, accounting for some 25–30 per cent of all cases. Being such a relatively large group it is possible to define syndromes within it—notably one with a peculiar chromosome abnormality involving chromosomes number 8 and 21 that shows a more favourable response to treatment.

The clinical picture that M2 AML presents is not dissimilar from M0/M1 AML. Occasionally the '8/21' variety can produce lumps of leukaemic cells outside the blood or marrow. These can vary from the size of a golf ball to a cricket ball, and can occasionally be discovered in that way before bone marrow failure becomes apparent. Such lumps, called *chloromas* because they have a greenish hue when surgically removed and cut in two (*chloros* = green), are usually found round the eye socket, brain, or spinal cord. They come to light either because they cause pain or because they cause a visible swelling.

## M3 AML

Also called *acute promyelocytic leukaemia*, M3 AML is perhaps the most distinctive and clearly defined subtype of AML. It is a rare disease in children accounting for around 10 per cent of the total, or one case in 100 of all childhood leukaemias. It is distinctive for two reasons. First, the leukaemic blast cells have a very characteristic appearance and are quite recognizable as immature neutrophils, albeit with some abnormal features. Some are packed with bundles of Auer

Rods (see above). Secondly the disease is regularly associated with a vicious bleeding tendency which is worse than that seen in other types of leukaemia.

The bleeding tendency is caused not only by a lack of platelets but also an additional lack of plasma clotting chemicals. These are lacking because the M3 blast cells contain and release powerful enzymes capable of digesting blood clotting proteins in the plasma. Following the start of chemotherapy, widespread disruption of the leukaemic cells can lead to a sudden worsening of the bleeding problem with a high risk of serious internal haemorrhage—especially into the brain, which can, of course, be rapidly fatal. If the initial problems of bleeding can be overcome, patients with M3 AML have a more favourable outlook (see below).

M3 disease also carries an almost invariable and highly specific chromosome abnormality in the malignant cells involving chromosomes numbers 15 and 17. This abnormality may give a clue to the cause of the disorder, because cells that have it fail to bind to their surface a vitamin A derivative, *trans*-retinoic acid, that is involved in controlling cell growth. Giving this substance in abnormally large doses can get round the problem to some extent, and can allow the M3 blasts to mature into (abnormal but harmless) neutrophils. It does not cure the disease, but can get patients gently into remission and avoid the danger of uncontrolled bleeding seen with conventional chemotherapy. This novel approach to the treatment of leukaemia is so far unique, but may be a way forward in other disorders when more about cell growth and maturation is understood.

There are no particular symptoms and signs other than those relating to extensive bruising that distinguish M3 disease from M0–2.

## M4 and M5 AML

These two leukaemias are hallmarked by the fact that both involve *immature monocytes*. The first (M4) is a hybrid where some of the blast cells show features of immature monocytes and some of immature neutrophils, and the second (M5) is true-bred where all the cells show a single lineage of early stage monocytes. The first is also called *acute myelomonocytic* leukaemia, and the second *acute monocytic* (or *monoblastic*) leukaemia. Together they account for about 15 per cent of AMLs in children.

Like all AMLs, monocytic leukaemias can arise at any age, but the M5 variant shows a predilection for very early infancy and can even rarely be present at birth. Very young babies with M5 AML often show patches of leukaemic cells under the skin which appear as flat raised firm spots with a dusky red colour about the size of peas or small beans. In older children, with teeth, both M4 and M5 AML can also be associated with impressive swelling of the gums. This is an unusual finding among the leukaemias and can be diagnostically helpful.

Monocyte-related AMLs also have a higher incidence of infiltration into the spinal fluid, and can produce symptoms such as headaches and vomiting, otherwise the features at presentation can be indistinguishable from other types of AML. There are some specific chromosome changes associated with some subtypes of M4/M5 AML, but so far only one, involving chromosome 16, has any major importance in terms of treatment response or outlook (see below).

## M6 AML (erythroleukaemia)

Leukaemias involving just immature early red cells are extremely rare in children and account for only 1–2 per cent of AMLs. Early developing red cells do not have the haemoglobin in them that makes them coloured, so the malignant blasts can look much like any other leukaemic cells, and no different in colour.

With M6 disease it is common to find that the developing neutrophils are involved in the disease process as well, so it is often a 'mixed' leukaemia. Looked at the other way round, it is not unusual to see abnormal developing red cells (a few) in M1/M2 AML, so the distinction of M6 from other types of AML is not always as clear cut as might be supposed. It is based on the *proportion* of malignant cells that are derived from red cells, and only when these are the dominant type of blast is the leukaemia classified as M6. The clinical picture and course of M6 AML is essentially similar to M0/M1/M2 AML.

## M7 AML (megakaryoblastic leukaemia)

The leukaemia derived from the third major bone marrow cell production line, that producing platelets, involves the earliest cell in that line, the *megakaryoblast*. Megakaryoblasts (normal sized cells) mature into megakaryocytes which break up to form platelets as described in Chapter 3. Megakaryocytes are the largest cells in the body and contain more than the usual amount of DNA. They are very easy to recognize. Megakaryoblasts, on the other hand, are fairly featureless cells that cannot easily be distinguished from immature neutrophils (or even lymphocytes). They are best recognized by specially made antibodies that identify cell features unique to platelets. For this reason M7 AML can only be confidently diagnosed using immunological techniques.

M7 AML is the only type of AML that is commoner in children than in adults. Children with Down syndrome are peculiarly susceptible to it in their early years, but it also occasionally arises in normal children. It sometimes presents in much the same way as other types of AML with bruising, infections, and pallor, but not infrequently its onset is more insidious with only small numbers of blast cells in the bloodstream. Bone marrow can be very difficult to obtain because there is an excess of tough scar-like tissue inside the marrow cavity (stimulated by the malignant cells in some way), and this can hinder the diagnosis. More commonly than other types of spontaneous (as opposed to secondary) AML, M7 disease can be preceded by a period of deranged bone marrow function and blood cytopenias forming a myelodysplastic syndrome (see Chapter 14).

## Secondary AML

One of the unpleasant paradoxes of anti-cancer chemotherapy is that some of the drugs used can themselves cause malignant disease, and the commonest expression of this capability is secondary AML. The drugs that do this are of two broad categories, the *alkylating agents* and the *topoisomerase II inhibitors*. Examples of the former include *cyclophosphamide*, *melphalan*, *mustine*, and *busulphan*. Examples of the latter include *etoposide* and *teniposide*, together with the anthracyclines *doxorubicin* and *epirubicin*. The type of leukaemia produced by these two categories of drug differs.

Alkylating drugs damage cells in the marrow and can cause genetic corruption particularly in chromosomes numbers 5 and or 7. There may be a long period where the bone marrow does not function properly giving rise to anaemia or other low blood counts but without evidence of frank leukaemia. The leukaemia that follows is usually of type M1 or M2. The process takes from 3 to 8 years after exposure to the drug. The problem was first recognized in survivors of Hodgkin's disease, a cancer of the lymphatic glands where alkylating agents have been a cornerstone of treatment. Secondary leukaemia occurred in 2–4 per cent of patients. Avoidance of such heavy use of alkylating agents has reduced the frequency of the problem.

Topoisomerase II inhibitors cause a different type of genetic corruption in marrow cells, involving chromosome 11 at a specific point—band 23 on the long arm, referred to as 11q23. This causes a mutation in the *mixed lineage leukaemia* (*mll*) gene. The leukaemia that follows has a shorter incubation time of 2–3 years, and the problem was seen in a small proportion of children (1–2 per cent) with ALL in one particular trial that relied heavily on teniposide. In this case the type of leukaemia is usually of type M4 or M5, involving the monocyte line.

Both types of secondary leukaemia are particularly difficult to treat as the response to conventional AML therapy is poor.

The next chapter describes the treatment of AML, the outcome, factors that influence outcome, and the management of relapse.

# Acute myeloid leukaemia (AML): current treatment schedules

Despite the availability of effective drugs for AML (cytarabine, anthracyclines, thioguanine) in the 1970s, at that time the results of treatment for both children and adults were dismal, with only 10–20 per cent becoming long-term disease-free survivors. Since then there has been dramatic progress in the outlook for both children and young adults, and it is true to say that in the last decade the improvement for children with AML has been more dramatic than that for children with ALL. It can now be claimed that over 50 per cent of childhood AML sufferers will survive their ordeal. In parallel with this advance has come the ability to categorize children into risk groups, like ALL, and this influences treatment decisions.

New drugs have become available since the 1970s and these have contributed to the better results of treatment, but the main factor has been the more effective use of existing agents and the design of schedules best described as based on the 'short sharp shock' philosophy. Unlike ALL, AML does not respond to long continual courses of drugs and maintenance treatment has no place. The approach is to use a combination of drugs in high doses over a few days to hit the disease hard, wait a week or two for the normal marrow to recover, then repeat the process with different drugs over four to six cycles. This gives a total treatment time of 4–6 months, very much shorter than the 2 years for ALL. Another major difference from ALL is that all the treatment has to be given in hospital and there is often little time at home during the chemotherapy programme due to the need for supportive measures (intravenous antibiotics, and blood and platelet transfusions) between courses.

Because the outlook was so poor, it used to be common practice to contemplate a bone marrow transplant in all patients who achieved remission after one or two courses. This is no longer so. The results of chemotherapy alone have now improved to the point where transplants are reserved for those in the less favourable risk groups (see below).

The drugs used include *cytarabine* (also called *cytosine arabinoside*), the two anthracyclines *adriamycin* and *daunorubicin* (the latter also called *rubidomycin* because of its bright red colour), *thioguanine*, and *etoposide*. They are described in Chapter 7 as they are all used in ALL as well. The doses and schedules in AML are different, however. Cytarabine, for example, is given at very high doses.

There are also other AML agents not routinely used in ALL. They include *mitoxantrone*, a compound closely related to the anthracyclines and distinguished by its vivid blue colour, and *amsacrine* (also known as M-AMSA), a drug with a similar action to the anthracyclines but a different chemical constitution. In addition drugs are used that potentiate the effect of high-dose cytarabine, *fludarabine* and *L-asparaginase* (the latter is the same drug as used in the treatment of ALL but employed here in a different role to alter the chemical behaviour of cells).

The drugs used to treat AML depress normal bone marrow production and cause profound bone marrow failure. Their main side-effects revolve round this, and it limits the doses that can be used. Most also produce nausea and vomiting, and loss of hair. With the exception of thioguanine, all agents have to be injected, and many are highly unpleasant substances that can cause skin blisters or tissue burns if not injected directly into the patient's bloodstream and diluted. Amsacrine cannot be given in plastic syringes as it dissolves the plastic. Glass must be used. Fludarabine is an extraordinary suppressor of immunity and special precautions need to be taken when using it.

AML does very occasionally involve the central nervous system (CNS, the brain and spinal cord), but with much less frequency than ALL. For this reason, as a precaution, it is usual to give one or two lumbar punctures and to inject a combination of methotrexate, cytarabine, and steroids. Most children's cancer centres would not pursue CNS-directed treatment any further than that and would avoid radiation treatment unless there were obvious blast cells in the spinal fluid at the time of diagnosis.

# Clinical trials and treatment programmes

As with ALL, much of the progress in AML has been as a result of national collaborative clinical trials where experimental treatments have been carefully assessed simultaneously in many children's cancer centres. Detailed results have been pooled and painstakingly analysed to learn about the best drug combinations, how to avoid complications and how to deal with side-effects. Presently there is much public concern about clinical trials and how well informed parents and children in them actually are about what is happening to them. This is understandable, and while every effort is made to explain fully why trials are needed and what is involved, it is often difficult for families struggling to cope with a life-threatening illness to appreciate the detailed rationale and technical aspects of trial questions.

Because of this difficulty some of the most important questions cannot be answered in the context of a proper randomized trial, and an important example is defining the role of bone marrow transplantation in AML. For children with good risk AML (see below) the current consensus is that transplantation probably offers no advantage (but this is not certain). For those with poor risk resistant disease there is little to lose, but for the bulk of patients who fall into neither category, we simply do not know which children will benefit from a transplant and which will not need such a potentially risky and damaging procedure. A clear case for a randomized trial, but one that will never be done.

The problem is that the concept of allocating such a major procedure on the toss of a coin leaves patients and parents (and often doctors) too uncomfortable to agree and they understandably refuse to participate. This means that insufficient numbers would be accumulated to give a reliable answer to the question. The only alternative is the accumulation of anecdotal evidence ('we tried transplantation in one group of patients and they seemed to do well, but the other group did not') which is less reliable and prone to misleading bias.

Despite these difficulties, successful trials of different drug combinations have been carried out in childhood AML. The current United Kingdom study is examining whether there is any advantage in five courses of combination chemotherapy over four. Bone marrow transplantation is an option for all children who do not fall into the favourable risk group, and whether or not children actually receive a transplant is based chiefly on the availability of a suitable donor (see Chapter 13).

# Treatment results and outlook in AML

The outlook for children with primary (as opposed to secondary) AML has improved to the point where currently around half can look forward to long-term leukaemia-free survival. Treatment failure, when it occurs, is of two types; first where the disease either fails to respond or responds initially with subsequent relapse, or secondly where the patient fails to survive the treatment and dies of some complication of bone marrow failure or other drug side-effect. Presently, about 10 per cent of patients have disease resistant to the drugs used, 35 per cent have disease that responds initially and then relapses, and 10 per cent fall by the wayside with death related to the treatment rather than the disease.

## Risk factors

The likelihood of death related to the treatment, a greater consideration than for ALL, depends, of course, on what the treatment is and the state of health of the patient. But let us first consider the risk of non-response, or initial response with later relapse.

As with ALL, the only real risk factor is therapy, without which the disease is 100 per cent fatal. But since the same treatment is given to children with all types of AML, it is possible to search for patterns of response relating to disease features (such as particular chromosome abnormalities) in an attempt to spot those that do better and those that do worse than average.

For AML, in contrast to ALL, there is no clear relationship between the white cell count, age, or sex and response to treatment, though very high white counts put patients at risk of circulatory failure through making the circulating blood too sticky to get through vital organs like the brain. There are, however, some differences in outcome for those with different leukaemic cell chromosome abnormalities. Also important is the speed of response to treatment.

### Favourable chromosomes

Children with M2 AML where there is a swap of DNA between chromosomes 8 and 21 do well, as do all children with M3 AML and the hallmark chromosome abnormality involving chromosomes 15 and 17. There is also a group of children with M4 AML who have DNA on chromosome 16 flipped upside down. They too respond better to treatment than other patients. Collectively these children, identified in the genetics laboratory, are regarded as 'good risk' with the best outlook and not as suitable candidates for the risks involved in bone marrow transplantation in their first remission. They stand a

70 per cent chance of long-term disease-free survival with chemo-therapy alone. Together they account for some 20 per cent of the total number of children with AML.

## Speed of response to treatment

Children without these abnormalities who nevertheless remit quickly after one course of treatment (like the fictitious Mary in Chapter 1) are regarded as 'standard risk' and all other patients are classified as 'high risk'. Around 70 per cent of AML children fall into the standard risk group and 10 per cent into the high risk category.

Given a first-remission bone marrow transplant from another individual (as opposed to an autologous transplant from themselves) long-term survival in childhood AML is of the order of 50 per cent in most centres, so, because the procedure carries a relatively high risk of death due to treatment-related complications, it is not presently considered to offer any advantage for good risk children and is reserved for the standard and poor risk groups.

## Down syndrome

Traditionally it was thought that the poor infants with Down syndrome who developed AML did particularly badly, and this was put down to their weak constitutions rather than the indolent nature of their leukaemias, but that may have been a problem of approach. If they are treated as other patients their response and treatment tolerance is similar enough to justify such an approach and that the overall outlook for those surviving therapy is relatively good.

## Other predisposing diseases

Other children predisposed to develop primary AML (see Chapter 14) may also be no different from normal in their response to treatment, though some, whose underlying disease is associated with peculiarly fragile chromosomes (those with *Fanconi's anaemia* or *Bloom's syndrome*, very rare conditions) are exquisitely sensitive to anti-cancer drugs and therefore are hard to treat as aggressively as normal children.

## Secondary AML

Perhaps the best defined poor risk group of AML patients is those with any form of secondary AML. Their response to treatment is invariably inferior. The problem is that they either fail to remit or relapse very quickly if they do. The results of bone marrow transplantation are not much more encouraging.

### Treatment-related deaths

Part of the problem of defining high risk AML patients is that treatment-related deaths can arise in those with the most responsive types of disease and confuse the picture.

As well as bone marrow failure which causes profound neutropenia and predisposes to septicaemia (see Chapter 12), damage can occur to other organs, notably the intestines. The lining of the intestines is delicate and composed of cells that have a high death and replacement rate in normal circumstances. Following intensive chemotherapy that lining can become damaged, the bowel can break down, perforate, and allow bacteria that normally live there harmlessly to escape from inside the bowel into the bloodstream or into the outer lining of the bowel called the *peritoneum* causing a serious infection (*peritonitis*) with pain and loss of bowel function. There can also be blood loss into or around the bowel, and this can sometimes be catastrophic.

A related and sinister problem that can arise in any patient with neutropenia and leukaemia (ALL or AML) is caused by inflammation and infection within the bowel wall, particularly at the junction where the long thin food-absorbing small intestine widens out into the waste matter-processing large bowel or colon. The appendix is positioned at this site, so the pain caused by *neutropenic colitis* (as the syndrome is called) is similar, at least to begin with, to appendicitis. Neutropenic colitis (sometimes also called *typhlitis*) can progress to peritonitis and can cause a blockage in the bowel leading to persistent vomiting and fluid loss. Surgery is not usually helpful. The only effective treatment is antibiotics, platelet transfusions (to prevent internal bleeding), and total parenteral nutrition to take over the function of the intestines while they are unable to work. Once neutrophils start to reappear, the condition usually improves quite rapidly, but before that stage is reached, a small number of sufferers will perish despite supportive therapy.

# Relapse of AML: treatment and outcome

Relapse of AML of any type is a very serious development and the chances of successful 'salvage' therapy are extremely slim at present.

Those patients who have not had any type of transplant should be urgently considered for one if a second remission can be achieved with further courses of aggressive treatment. Those relapsing after a transplant may be eligible for donor lymphocyte infusions (see Chapter 13). Like ALL, patients relapsing a long time off therapy fare better in terms of incidence and duration of second remissions, but there are far fewer long survivors.

Where aggressive therapy is inappropriate, sometimes reasonable palliative disease control can be achieved for a few weeks or months using low-dose domiciliary injections of cytarabine coupled with oral thioguanine. An alternative is daily oral low-dose etoposide.

# 12

# Supportive treatment for children with leukaemia

Many problems beset children and their families when they try to come to terms with leukaemia and the difficulties of struggling through treatment. One thing is certain. Life will never be the same again.

Once the initial shock has started to subside and the treatment programme has got under way the main initial hurdles are medical—dealing with the side-effects and complications of chemotherapy. There is also (particularly for ALL) the problem of organizing the complicated drug schedules in a workable way that allows some sort of normal rhythm to return to everyday life. Most families cope magnificently. Some, particularly those where the course of the disease and treatment are unexpectedly stormy, have a more difficult time with stress-related psychological disorders arising in patients, parents, and brothers and sisters. These family difficulties are described in Chapter 15. The following section focuses on the practical problems of getting through the various treatment programmes.

## Central venous catheters

The now near universal use of some sort of central venous catheter in all children being treated for any type of acute leukaemia has made life very much easier for everyone concerned. These catheters are thin plastic tubes pushed under the skin of the chest, tunnelled over the outside of the ribs and inserted into a large vein directly above the heart. Insertion requires an anaesthetic and a minor operation. The procedure is usually carried out in the first few days following diagnosis.

The catheter is stitched in place and can be repeatedly attached and unattached to syringes, pumps, or gravity drip infusions with ease.

It is sometimes referred to as a *central line* or called after the particular model design such as *Hickman*, *Broviac* or *Groshong*. Some lines have more than one barrel, useful if intensive supportive treatment involving more than one thing at once might be needed such as following bone marrow transplantation.

There is a different type of appliance in which the entire device is under the skin. A small plastic resevoir is positioned on the chest wall into which needles can be pushed and from which a catheter leads into a vein like other central lines. This is commonly referred to as a *Portacath* (the brand name of one of the most popular models). It does not avoid the use of needles, but is otherwise easy to access and needs less looking after on a day-to-day basis. It only has one barrel.

Central lines are not without problems. They need scrupulous care to avoid them becoming infected, and they have to be regularly flushed to avoid them becoming blocked. Despite this blood clots and infections of the plastic tubes used are common. Clots and blockages need the injection of clot-dissolving drugs such as *urokinase* or anti-coagulants such as *heparin*. As for infections, bacteria are particularly good at colonizing these devices and can be quite hard to get rid of. If persistently present they present a threat to patients during periods of neutropenia, so powerful antibiotics need to be instilled into the catheter. If blockages, clots, and infections cannot be resolved by these means, the device has to be removed. A new one can be inserted on the opposite side, but usually on a separate occasion after a course of antibiotics.

# Complications of chemotherapy

## Bone marrow failure

All types of leukaemia have one thing in common. Untreated, they are lethal because they eventually cause complete bone marrow failure. This is described in Chapter 4. Bone marrow is just as much a vital organ as the heart, kidneys, or liver. If the function of the bone marrow (producing blood cells) is impaired serious problems result. If anyone has total and irreversible loss of function, they cannot survive for very long. When the marrow fails there is a lack of red blood cells, white blood cells, and platelets. This respectively causes anaemia, susceptibility to certain types of infection, and a bleeding tendency.

The paradox of leukaemia therapy is that the drugs used to treat it also cause bone marrow failure from time to time. It is the management of this problem that causes most of the need to attend hospital during remission between courses of chemotherapy and generates the demand for intravenous antibiotics, blood, and blood component transfusions.

Chemotherapy causes marrow failure in the same way as it kills leukaemia cells—by interfering with the process of cell division. The various drugs can be thought of as analogous to selective weed-killers. At the right dose they kill leukaemic cells but spare normal cells. Too little, and the leukaemic cells survive. Too much and normal cells die with the marrow being severely damaged. This explains why the doses are always pushed to the point where the marrow is damaged a little, but not to the point where it cannot recover after a few days rest. The marrow is the most vulnerable normal tissue because it is the organ with the highest rate of cell division. The next most vulnerable organ is the intestine, and the lining of the bowels can also become damaged by chemotherapy, particularly the high doses used to treat AML or following preparatory therapy for bone marrow transplantation (see *neutropenic colitis*, Chapter 11).

It is helpful to consider the management of marrow failure under the three categories of anaemia, lack of platelets, and lack of white cells.

## Anaemia

Failure to produce sufficient red cells or loss of red cells through bleeding or premature destruction in the body can lead to a fall in the blood concentration of haemoglobin (commonly referred to as Hb) below normal. The main cause of anaemia during therapy for leukaemia is the suppression of red cell production by chemotherapy. This can be temporarily corrected by transfusing haemoglobin-containing red cells from a blood donor. The transfused cells will survive for a few weeks, usually sufficient to tide a child over until the normal marrow function kicks in again. Transfusing red cells in this way is what is loosely referred to as a 'blood transfusion' but in truth is only a blood *component* transfusion as the white cells, platelets, and much of the plasma will have been removed.

Red cells for transfusion are selected on the basis of the appropriate blood group. Blood groups were unknown until the beginning of the twentieth century. Before that the fact that sometimes person-to-person transfusions of blood seemed to work and sometimes they killed patients remained a source of frustration. Then a young

Viennese scientist called Karl Landsteiner discovered that the serum (plasma with the clotting chemicals taken out) from some individuals contained the ability to make red cells from some others stick together in clumps (*agglutinate*). This is a process quite distinct and different from coagulation. The pattern of agglutination between individuals led him to suggest that there were three blood groups, which he called A, B, and C. Later in a larger study a fourth rare group was discovered. It was called group AB, and group C was renamed group O. The substances in the serum causing cell clumping turned out to be *antibodies*, and these were recognizing corresponding A and B *antigens* on the red cells.

Life is never simple, and after the ABO groups were discovered it was not long before other 'families' of antigens on red cells, different from those of the ABO groups and relating to other (less important) blood group systems were discovered. The most well known is the *Rhesus* system.

What is most important when transfusing red cells from a donor to a recipient is *whether the recipient has antibodies to the donor's red cells*. Donor blood for transfusion is laboratory tested against the serum of any intended recipients to make sure that they do not. The test is called a *cross-match*. Laboratories nowadays may simply screen the recipient's serum for the presence of any antibodies rather than do a full cross-match donor by donor. Normally only antibodies to ABO antigens are present, but patients who have had previous transfusions (or pregnancies) may have developed others.

When otherwise healthy marrow is suppressed by chemotherapy, the red cells usually disappear slowly over a time scale of several days or weeks. Rapid disappearance indicates that there is cell destruction or loss, otherwise they vanish at the rate of 1–2 per cent a day. There is no magic level of blood haemoglobin that prompts an automatic transfusion. The need for red cells is assessed on how the child is and whether the Hb is rising or falling as well as the actual measured concentration.

## Lack of platelets (thrombocytopenia)

Platelets disappear more quickly than red cells if their production is stopped. The prime function of these strange little cells is to patrol the circulatory system and maintain the integrity of the pipes and tubes by plugging small leaks and helping blood to clot where larger holes appear. A good test of how they are working and whether there are enough is to make a small nick in the skin and see how long it takes to stop bleeding. Platelets are destroyed in the process of being called into service at the site of a leak and so the rate of disappearance when the marrow is suppressed is rather variable. The time to achieve low counts varies from a day in patients who are sick and bleeding to a week or more in children who are otherwise well.

Problems through lack of platelets seldom arise until the number in the circulation falls below 5–10 per cent of normal. Even at that stage there may be no sign of the problem in well children. Exactly when platelets should be transfused depends on the clinical circumstances and the local policy of the unit concerned. Some physicians transfuse in all circumstances when the platelet count falls below a threshold to prevent rather than to treat bleeding. Others do so only in circumstances when bleeding is more likely or where it is known that the platelets will disappear completely for a while (such as following marrow transplantation). Everyone transfuses platelets in the face of active bleeding in a child with a very low platelet count.

Platelet transfusions are different from red cell transfusions. They carry the same blood group characteristics as red cells so usually only platelets of a suitable ABO group are used. They also carry some of the more complicated group characteristics of white cells (see tissue types, Chapter 13) and can occasionally be rapidly destroyed if a patient has antibodies to these tissue groups. In that event especially compatible tissue-matched platelets may be needed, but these are in short supply so are not used routinely.

The material actually transfused is either a pool of platelets harvested from four or five routine blood donations or platelets from a single donor harvested on a machine called a cell separator. Here blood is taken out of one arm, the platelets are removed with some plasma, and the remainder of the blood is returned to the other arm in a continuous flow. This process is known as *apheresis*. The platelets are spun and filtered to remove unwanted white and red cells, and appear as a slightly cloudy straw coloured fluid.

Transfused platelets normally survive a few days in well children. In sick children they may be rapidly consumed, and they may also disappear rapidly if the recipient has developed antibodies to them and thus become refractory. Because of the latter problem it is best to be as economical with platelet transfusions as possible so that they do not lose their beneficial effect at a time when they are needed most.

## Lack of white cells

Because of the different types, lack of white cells is rather more complicated than lack of red cells or platelets. In one way or another all white cells are involved with defending the body against invasion or infection, but they do this in different ways and have different roles against different invaders. There are only two types that are vital for survival and these are not equally affected by chemotherapy, which further complicates the issue.

### Neutrophils

Neutrophils are the most numerous white cells in the blood of healthy children over the age of 4. Not only are they the most frequent cells, but they are also the most sensitive to chemotherapy, and, having a short life span, disappear within a day or two of a major onslaught on the marrow such as the courses of treatment used for AML. They also recover the most quickly

### Lymphocytes

Lymphocytes are the second commonest white cell and are less sensitive to 'short sharp shock' type chemotherapy but gradually become suppressed by the long drawn-out maintenance phase of treatment for ALL. They take several weeks or months to recover full function.

Anything that damages the body's defences against infection causes a patient to be described as *immunosuppressed* or *immunocompromised*. These terms are used loosely but do not define a precise state. The consequences of lack of neutrophils (*neutropenia*) are different from those of a lack of lymphocytes (*lymphopenia*). To understand how they differ it is important to appreciate the broad categories of infection.

## Types of infection

Infection is the successful invasion of the body by a micro-organism (the terms germ or bug are colloquial alternatives) which multiplies and thrives at the expense of the host. Such invaders are divided into the broad categories of bacteria, viruses, and fungi. Bacteria are cellular organisms that consist of a single cell. They multiply by simply dividing, like all cells. Most do not cause disease, and billions live quietly on the skin and in the intestines of every healthy human. Viruses are not cellular, but consist of an aggregate of chemicals that

enter human cells, reproduce there, and then emerge, usually destroy-
ing the cell in the process. Some are carried within the body without
causing disease because they are prevented from multiplying. They
are smaller than bacteria and only the very largest can be seen with
ordinary microscopes. Fungi are composed of single or several cells,
depending on the type. They seldom cause serious disease in healthy
people though can cause irritating problems. In immunosuppressed
patients, on the other hand, they can be lethal.

Well known bacterial infections include boils, meningitis, acute
bronchitis, and tooth abscesses. Well known virus infections include
the common cold, warts, influenza, measles, chicken pox, and AIDS.
Common fungal infections include athlete's foot and thrush.

## Infection and neutropenia

Children who are neutropenic are particularly vulnerable to bacteria
and fungi. This means that during episodes when the neutrophil
count is very low there is a risk of normally relatively harmless bacteria gaining access to the body and multiplying in the bloodstream
unchecked. This is called *septicaemia* (*sepsis* = infection, *aemia* = in
the blood). The source of such bacteria is usually the child's own skin
or intestine. Prolonged neutropenia can also allow normally harmless
fungi to gain access to the deep tissues in the body and cause serious
infections, particularly in the lungs and liver.

### Fever and neutropenia

Because of this risk, children with neutropenia who develop signs of
possible infection, usually a rise in body temperature (a fever), are
treated immediately with powerful intravenous antibiotics while a
search is made for bacteria in the bloodstream and elsewhere. Often,
fever in neutropenic children is not associated with a bacterial infection and is probably due to a relatively trivial virus infection, but this
cannot reliably be assumed and that is why the problem is taken so
seriously.

It is important to stress that 'neutropenia' in this context means a
neutrophil count of less than 10 per cent of the lower limit of normal,
and that a few neutrophils are usually enough to keep patients out of
trouble. The type of antibiotics used in fever with neutropenia
depend on the policy of the unit concerned, the likely source of infection if known (such as a central venous catheter, see below), and
whether any bacteria have been identified in the laboratory. It is very

rare for a serious infection to prove fatal because of the wrong choice of antibiotics, and in truth it probably matters less which drugs are used than that treatment with something with a wide spectrum of anti-bacterial activity is used as quickly as is reasonably possible.

Fungal infections can cause fever in neutropenic children but usually the problem creeps up in patients already on antibiotics for possible bacterial infection. Normal antibiotics are no use against fungi and special drugs have to be used. These are often given on suspicion of fungal infection rather than proof, and sometimes are given to prevent fungal infection occurring in the first place.

### Growth factors

To shorten the period of post-intensive chemotherapy neutropenia, sometimes the neutrophil growth factor G-CSF (see Chapter 4) is given, and similarly it may become common practice to use thrombopoietin to shorten the period of low platelet counts. The difference these compounds make is not dramatic, but they can successfully minimize the period of risk from bleeding and infection. G-CSF (or GM-CSF, see Chapter 4) is quite widely used because there is no alternative way of increasing the neutrophil count. They may drive the neutrophils to reappear 1 or 2 days earlier than otherwise would be the case. Platelets and red cells can be transfused, so there is perhaps less need for thrombopoietin or erythropoietin in this setting.

## Infection and lymphopenia

The lymphocyte count does not have such a clear-cut relationship with infection problems as the neutrophil count. Some children may have problems resisting certain types of infection irrespective of the numbers of circulating lymphocytes; if so they demonstrate suppressed lymphocyte *function*. The problem is more or less confined to two groups of patients in the context of childhood leukaemia—those on maintenance treatment for ALL and those in the first few months following bone marrow transplantation. Both tend to have low lymphocyte counts but both also have defective lymphocyte function.

Maintenance treatment for ALL predisposes to infections where lymphocyte function is important—mostly viruses but also an unusual type of pneumonia also seen in AIDS patients caused by a strange organism called *Pneumocystis carinii* thought to be related to fungi. *Pneumocystis* pneumonia is now rarely seen because children at risk are given a specific antibiotic (co-trimoxazole, trade name Septrin or

Bactrim) two or three times each week, which provides excellent protection. Before this was done *Pneumocystis* used regularly to claim a few lives of children in remission from their leukaemia.

Two other potentially troublesome invaders for children with defective lymphocyte function are the viruses causing chickenpox and measles.

## Chickenpox

Because chickenpox is widespread, and because it is not considered serious enough to warrant a routine immunization programme, many children will have had the disease before they ever develop leukaemia. They, like all who have had it, will then have the virus with them for ever. It hibernates quietly deep inside the body and only flares up if the person becomes old, run down, or otherwise debilitated. When it flares up, it usually (but not always) confines itself to one small part of the body, commonly the trunk, or head, or neck. Such a recurrent attack is called *shingles* or *zoster* and produces the well known and often painful rash. Occasionally a reactivated attack can be generalized and look like a new infection with spots all over. Chickenpox and shingles are thus both manifestations of the same virus (called *varicella-zoster*).

New infection (the classic chickenpox, more correctly called *varicella*) is the result of contact with active disease (i.e. fresh spots)—either chickenpox or shingles. Such contact needs to be more than just being in the same room and usually involves physical touching. Old infection flaring up represents the already present virus being reactivated and is not the result of contact with an active case. It is important to remember that once children have had chickenpox they cannot catch it again because they never get rid of it.

A new or reactivated attack of varicella-zoster can usually be stopped in its tracks by a drug called *acyclovir*, but a bad attack of the disease will need this to be given in hospital and intravenously. Usually the problem can be controlled in this way, and it is not the scourge of children with ALL that it once was, though very rare fatalities do still occur.

When susceptible children who have never had chickenpox before are in very close (touching or playing) contact with an active case of chickenpox or shingles (non-crusted spots), steps can be taken to try to prevent such patients catching the disease. They can either be given an injection of a specially prepared form of blood plasma containing high concentrations of antibodies to the virus (*zoster immune globulin* or ZIG), or given a course of acyclovir by mouth for 3 weeks to cover the incubation phase of the disease.

It is very important, however, to keep the chickenpox risk in perspective. It is a widespread disease always present in the community, and cases are cropping up in schools and playgroups all the time. To deny leukaemia sufferers the pleasures of social contact with their peers to avoid the small risk of contact is indefensible.

### Measles

Measles is much more of a worry than chickenpox because there is no specific therapy, and a substantial proportion of leukaemia patients on maintenance treatment who get it may die. Fortunately it is a much, much more rare disease in developed countries, as nearly all babies are now immunized against it. Many younger paediatricians have never seen a case, and no children in the United Kingdom childhood ALL trials have been reported to have developed the disease in recent years.

Measles in a child with deficient lymphocyte function can produce a different picture from the classical fever, runny nose, and rash. It has no rash and usually begins with fever and a cough that then progresses to widespread inflammation of the lungs (pneumonia). Then there is either slow recovery or gradual failure of lung function leading to death. There is no known effective treatment other than supportive therapy (oxygen and antibiotics to prevent microbes other than the measles virus taking advantage of the situation). Measles can also attack the brain, producing fits, and even coma.

If a patient has had contact with a child who has *confirmed* measles, an antibody concentrate from normal blood donors (immunoglobulin) can be given in an attempt to prevent the infection, but it may not be effective.

## Nutritional support

Children undergoing intensive chemotherapy lose their appetite, suffer from nausea and vomiting (though this can usually be alleviated by special anti-sickness drugs), may get mouth ulcers and not unreasonably get to feel rather low. Their intestines may be damaged by the chemotherapy leading to loss of normal function. All of this can lead to poor nutrition and at a time when extra demands are being placed on nutritional reserve.

Much can be achieved by a relaxed approach to the problem, though it is one that naturally creates considerable parental anxiety. Simple tasty dietary supplements may help over a short period. The next stage is to use a fine plastic tube put into the stomach through the nose and down the gullet, and to use that to trickle in special dietary formulae to boost nutrition. If that fails, the last resort is intravenous feeding—called *total parenteral nutrition* or TPN. 'Parenteral' mean by-passing the enteric route, i.e. the normal intestines.

TPN can be given through a central venous catheter and can replace the entire nutritional requirements of an individual child. It is used as a routine after bone marrow transplantation and other situations where the treatment is known to damage the intestines and they need time to recover. It is also used occasionally in other children, but because of the great inconvenience and the need to stay in hospital all the time it is used as little as possible.

# Intensive care

Children who develop serious infections, whether neutropenic or not, can occasionally develop the complication of failure of vital organ function (lungs, kidneys, or heart for example) for which the special support offered by intensive care units is needed. These units can support failing organs by the use of sophisticated machines and drugs, together with close monitoring and 24-hour specialist nursing.

The same facilities are occasionally needed in some types of leukaemia at the start of treatment. This occurs when the chemical storm from massive leukaemia cell breakdown causes temporary problems with kidney function and also other organs. Intensive care may also be necessary when internal bleeding occurs or when any catastrophe arises that seriously threatens the body's vital functions.

The inexorable trend toward ever more intensive treatment schedules has increased the need for support of this type and all children with leukaemia should have ready access to intensive care facilities even though the large majority will never need them. They have no part to play in terminal care, and children with organ failure associated with incurable disease should be allowed to die without artificial life support.

# Shared care

Many children with leukaemia live far away from the specialist children's cancer unit where their treatment is planned and organized.

Attendance may involve long distances, slow journey times, or both. Also, because of the increasing complexity and labour intensity of treatment protocols, many children's cancer units are having logistic difficulty coping with the day-to-day administration of those programmes and have devolved more and more to paediatric units in hospitals nearer the homes of the families involved.

The point has now been reached in the United Kingdom where much of the supportive treatment for children with ALL described above (excluding TPN and intensive care) is carried out in local hospitals with the help of interested nurses, paediatricians, and haematologists. The system is referred to in Chapter 1. Not only is supportive care provided, but in many instances the bulk of maintenance chemotherapy is controlled by the shared care centres as well. This avoids a lot of travelling for the children concerned.

Different hospitals practice different 'levels' of shared care, depending on several factors including the enthusiasm and experience of the local team, the numbers of patients they deal with, and local geography. At the lowest, local hospitals can carry out blood counts, housekeep central venous catheters, and provide initial treatment for fever and neutropenia. At the highest, shared care centres can diagnose and treat uncomplicated ALL without actually referring the child to a more specialist centre, though they still work in close collaboration by registering the patient and sending samples for (for example) genetic analysis.

Shared care also occasionally helps with children with AML, though only for simple supportive treatment. The more intensive nature of the actual chemotherapy means that such patients spend most of their time in specialist children's cancer units. Similarly, shared care has little to offer bone marrow transplant recipients in the early days following discharge apart from local blood tests for the routine monitoring of medication and other simple supportive measures. This situation may change in the next few years.

# 13

# Bone marrow transplantation

To understand the rationale and problems surrounding transplantation of bone marrow, it is important to have a grasp of what normal marrow is and how it functions. This is described in Chapter 4, and the reader is strongly recommended to read that, and Chapter 3 about normal blood cells, as a prelude to what follows.

The idea of bone marrow transplantation is not new. Attempts were being made to make marrow cells from one individual grow in another during the 1940s, but early experiments were unsuccessful because of the peculiar problems relating to compatibility and rejection. The progress made in recent years owes more to understanding and avoidance of such problems, rather than the development of more sophisticated techniques of physically transplanting marrow. Actually carrying out the procedure itself is extremely simple, as will become clear.

## Terms used in marrow transplantation

There are some terms used in marrow transplantation that it is helpful to be clear about. An *allogeneic* or *homologous* transplant (sometimes abbreviated to *allograft* or *homograft*) is one from a genetically unidentical donor. This is the usual type of bone marrow transplant where a brother or sister is a donor. Sometimes other relatives, or, increasingly, unrelated donors are used. A *syngeneic* transplant is one from a genetically identical donor, i.e. an identical twin, only very occasionally an option in leukaemia sufferers.

An *autologous* transplant, also called *autotransplant* or *autograft* is not, strictly speaking, a transplant at all, as it describes the process where a patient's *own* marrow is removed to be used as a source of marrow for the same person later on. It might better be termed a bone marrow *replant*, but the term autotransplant is now in common usage.

Increasingly frequently the term '*progenitor cell transplant*' is used instead of bone marrow transplant. '*Progenitor*' in this context means cells that can re-seed the recipient's marrow and develop into blood cells. They are the vitally important 'stem' cells that can be found not only in the marrow of donors, but also (in very small numbers) circulating in the blood. They can therefore not only be obtained by collecting bone marrow, but also can be concentrated and collected from blood processed through a cell separator machine (in a process called 'apheresis' described in Chapter 12) and used instead of marrow. They can also be found in relatively large numbers in the blood from newborn babies left behind in the after-birth. This *cord blood* (obtained from the umbilical cord of the after-birth) can be collected and processed and the stem cells frozen down for future use of patients who do not have a suitable related donor.

So it is not necessary always to use marrow to carry out a 'marrow' transplant, and the alternative name reflects this. Custom and practice, however, dictates that 'bone marrow transplantation' is still loosely talked about whether using *peripheral blood stem cells* (PBSC) or *cord blood stem cells* (CBSC), and for the sake of clarity in this chapter BMT will be used in its broadest sense.

# How BMT differs from transplantation of other organs

There is a fundamental difference between the transplantation of bone marrow and that of other organs such as kidneys, livers, hearts, and lungs. In the latter cases, there is the physical removal of a pre-formed organ and its insertion into another body. Difficulties involved relate to the intricacy of the surgery involved (re-establishing the blood supply and other anatomical connections), the condition of the organ being transplanted, and the immune system of the recipient in terms of the likelihood of a wholesale rejection attack being launched on the newly inserted foreign tissue.

In the transfer of bone marrow, there is no surgery, no pre-formed organ, and if there is any rejection, it is the graft that tries to reject the recipient, rather than vice versa. This is because it is a few progenitor cells that are being transferred that will re-grow into marrow and a new immune system. They can simply be transfused into the bloodstream and will find their own way to the marrow. To allow them to survive and grow, the recipient's own marrow and immune system has first to be eradicated otherwise the delicate stem cells would be killed off rapidly and the graft would fail.

The transfused stem cells repopulate the marrow over a few weeks, so the graft grows slowly, unlike (say) a kidney, which starts to function immediately. Because the recipient's immune system has been wiped out before the graft, it is unusual for a marrow graft to be rejected in the way that a heart might be. But because the transferred blood and marrow cells also repopulate the recipient's immune system with that from the donor, there is the possibility that the new system might regard the whole of the recipient's body as foreign and try to reject it all. This *graft-versus-host* reaction is the reason that marrow transplantation has been fraught with difficulties over the years and why it is so important to find donors that are as compatible as possible.

# What marrow transplantation can be used for

Theoretically, any disease of the bone marrow or immune system, either inherited or acquired, can be cured if the diseased marrow can be removed and replaced by healthy marrow grown from stem cells from another individual. Practically speaking, since marrow transplantation is still a risky business from which a proportion of patients will perish even in the best hands, the procedure is reserved for life-threatening or serious life-shortening illnesses where the benefits clearly outweigh the risks. Apart from malignant disease, these include the primary failure of bone marrow (*aplastic anaemia*, where normal marrow function just fizzles out) and serious immune deficiency disorders. In these circumstances the transplant is replacing something that is absent or malfunctioning.

The idea behind marrow transplantation for leukaemia is also to replace what is lacking, but as a secondary phenomenon. The actual transplant is used to reinstate the marrow (and the immune system) destroyed by aggressive treatment given to eradicate the malignant disease. It is, in a sense, a rescue procedure from what would otherwise be lethal treatment—lethal by causing irreversible marrow damage. Conventional chemotherapy is limited by its toxic effect on normal marrow. If that ceases to be a worry (because marrow will be replaced by the transplant), much higher doses can be explored. The same is true of whole body deep X-ray treatment, which would also otherwise completely eradicate the bone marrow.

This simple rescue process was the initial rationale for BMT in leukaemia, but as experience grew it became clear that patients who had some graft-versus-host reaction ran less risk of their leukaemia ever returning than those who did not. This observation indicated that a graft-versus-leukaemia immune attack seemed to operate in parallel with the graft-versus-host reaction, and indeed this is now thought to be the case. The immune component of BMT is therefore very important in the eradication of leukaemia (see 'graft-versus-leukaemia effect' below).

# How an allogeneic marrow transplant for leukaemia is carried out—the practical steps and what happens

Carrying out an allogeneic marrow transplant is not technically difficult and requires no expensive special equipment. For the treatment of leukaemia, the following conditions have to be met and steps taken.

1. The decision to pursue a transplant as an option has to be taken (see 'Who needs it?' below). In many children with leukaemia the chances of long-term disease-free survival will be *reduced* by an allogeneic transplant while in others the chances of a successful outcome are too small to justify the considerable discomfort and distress involved, so the decision has to be taken with care.

2. A compatible donor has to be found. Compatibility (outside the context of identical twins) is, of course, a question of degree and ranges from not at all to almost completely. The best option is a matched brother or sister, though increasingly unrelated donors are being used. The less compatible the donor, the greater the risk of failure and fatality (see 'Compatibility', below).

3. The patient has to be in remission from leukaemia. Although early patients were transplanted in the late and advanced stages of their disease, the results were very disappointing and many were subjected to what would now be regarded as unnecessary suffering. For the best chance of success, children should be well, have normal blood counts at the outset, and their disease should be under stable control.

4. The donor has to be willing and medically fit to undergo a general anaesthetic and blood loss equivalent of up to two full blood donations from an adult. Alternatively the donor has to be willing and old enough to be subjected to apheresis.

5. Before beginning, the recipient must have an indwelling central venous catheter (described in Chapter 12). This will be needed for transfusion of fluids, red cells, platelets, drugs, and intravenous feeding in the immediate post-transplant period. The catheter should therefore be one of the double- or triple-barrelled variety, allowing the infusion of more than one thing at once.

6. At the start, the patient and donor are both given a thorough medical examination to make sure that all is well.

7. The patient is admitted to hospital for the pre-transplant treatment. This is called the 'conditioning' treatment, and is referred to in a way that implies it to be simply to prepare the way for the transplant, but, as indicated above, for the child with leukaemia it is designed to do more than that. It is the treatment that will, hopefully, eradicate the bulk of his or her remaining blast cells. If inadequate or unsuccessful, it might leave sufficient malignant disease to survive the graft-versus-leukaemia effect and lead to post-transplant relapse.

For children undergoing bone marrow transplants for *non*-malignant diseases, the conditioning treatment is just that. It is for a different job—to prevent the recipient rejecting the transplant. For this reason the approach may be different.

For leukaemia sufferers, it is common practice to give a massive dose of a cytotoxic drug (commonly *cyclophosphamide*) on two successive days, followed by a course of whole body deep X-ray treatment, either all in one go, or, more usually, in instalments over 3 or 4 days. Children under 2 are not given radiation treatment, but usually receive a second cytotoxic drug as an alternative (often *busulphan*, a powerful marrow suppressant commonly used in much lower doses to control an adult type of chronic leukaemia). There is a growing trend to avoid total body radiation in young children because of the late side effects on growth (see Chapter 16), but it is still the standard approach. Sometimes other drug combinations are used, but doses are always much higher than those used conventionally. All conditioning schedules are capable of producing irreversible bone marrow failure, which is, after all, the idea.

8. At the end of the patient's conditioning treatment, the marrow is collected from the donor. This procedure is known as 'harvesting' bone marrow. It involves the donor being fully anaesthetized and taken into an operating theatre with full sterile precautions. With the donor lying on an operating table, bone marrow is sucked out of the hip bones through stout hollow needles about the diameter of knitting

needles. The material obtained looks like blood (and indeed *is* mostly blood) with a fatty scum on the top, and has to be kept from clotting by thorough mixing with anti-coagulants. It is collected into a bag like that used to collect blood donations, under strict sterile conditions.

The amount removed depends on how rich the material is in white cells and how big the intended recipient is. It is common practice, based on experience rather than theory, to obtain sufficient to provide the donor with around $3 \times 10^8$ marrow cells for each kilogram of his or her body weight. There is nothing magic in that figure, and perfectly successful transplants have been achieved with considerably less. Easily harvested healthy marrow contains around $5 \times 10^8$ cells in every 25 millilitres (5 teaspoons full). If the marrow is to be processed before being given to the recipient (see 9 below), more cells should be taken as some will be lost.

It is perhaps worth remembering that the crude unprocessed material removed from the marrow cavity of the hip bone is, in terms of what is needed for a successful transplant, something approaching 99 per cent unwanted material. It is the few precious stem cells that matter, but it is neither easy nor necessary to go to great lengths to isolate them.

If the donor is the same size or larger than the recipient, it is possible that the amount of marrow harvested can be tolerated without the need for a transfusion to replace lost red cells. If, though, the harvested marrow is not rich in cells (necessitating the taking of more for the same cell count) or the donor is a younger and smaller sibling of the recipient, the red cell loss may need to be replaced by a blood transfusion to avoid discomfort. Sometimes the donor's own blood, taken earlier, is re-transfused to avoid the risks of blood from another individual.

The procedure is usually complete in from 1 to 2 hours. The donor is allowed home the following morning, and will feel stiff and sore around the hips for a couple of days, otherwise there are usually no after-effects. Apart from the occasional need for red cell replacement transfusion, there is no change in the donor blood counts, and the lost marrow is made up almost immediately.

If marrow from an unrelated donor is being used, the donor may live many miles away or in a different country. In that case the marrow is harvested in a hospital near the donor's home and then transported as rapidly as possible to the recipient. If cord blood is being used, it is thawed out immediately before being given to the recipient.

9. The marrow is then given to the recipient. Depending on the type of donor (sibling or unrelated), and the custom and practice of the unit involved, it may be given straight from the harvest bag, or may be treated first to remove the red cells and/or some of the unwanted white cells. Either way, it is usually given immediately or within a few hours, and administered by simply running it slowly into a vein in exactly the same way as a transfusion of any other blood product and with no more fuss. The process of 'transplantation' is thus an intravenous infusion, and involves no surgery at all for the recipient.

The marrow stem cells, indistinguishable in their appearance from normal white blood cells, then circulate in the blood and leave the bloodstream on reaching a suitable environment—the recipient's bone marrow cavity, empty and waiting like a freshly dug flower bed with no plants in it. There they quietly go about the business of repopulating the marrow over the next few weeks and regenerating the recipient's immune system over the next few months. The transplant is over, but there are still plenty of things that can go wrong.

10. The pre-engraftment phase then follows during which time the recipient is kept in hospital. Before the new marrow starts to grow, the recipient's blood counts will tumble to zero, and there will be a period of profound bone marrow failure. Transfusions of platelets and red cells are usually needed. Care must be taken to avoid infection (as during any period of marrow failure), and for that reason many centres take elaborate precautions keeping transplant recipients in strict isolation in specially built cubicles with positive pressure ventilation to avoid extraneous micro-organisms drifting in. A few units arguably take things to ridiculous extremes, irradiating with gamma rays any items going into isolation cubicles to sterilize them, and severely restricting visitors, keeping them behind glass panels. Other units are more relaxed in their approach, and there is no evidence that their patients fare any worse.

During this time it is important to prevent graft-versus-host disease (see below). There are several different approaches to the problem. Sometimes the marrow itself is processed before the transplant to remove some of the T lymphocytes responsible for the immediate graft-versus-host reaction, and/or drugs are used that paradoxically suppress immunity and allow the new system slowly to 'recognize' the recipient as 'self'. The agents most frequently used are *methotrexate*, an anti-leukaemia drug but given in this context to stop normal donor lymphocytes dividing, and *cyclosporin*, a drug originally derived from a fungus that inhibits the function of T lymphocytes. It is also used to prevent organ transplants such as kidneys and hearts from being rejected. Most children's transplant centres now use cyclosporin alone. The drug is continued for a few months. Occasionally other drugs are used.

Nutrition may cause difficulties during the pre-engraftment and the early engraftment phase. The chemotherapy and total body deep X-ray schedule usually temporarily damages the lining of the intestines—a tissue that, like bone marrow, normally has a high cell turnover. This can produce nausea and diarrhoea, and often means that food cannot be absorbed, even if the child feels like eating. It is common practice to give a period of intravenous feeding to circumvent the problem.

The prevention of infection is paramount, but the source of the infections that trouble transplant recipients is often themselves. The organisms involved are ubiquitous and often carried harmlessly in normal healthy individuals. A particular concern is *cytomegalovirus* or CMV which can already be in the recipient or transferred from the donor (there is no way to avoid this if the donor is CMV-positive). In immunosuppressed post-transplant patients this can cause a severe and fatal disease with organ failure ivolving the lungs and liver. Antiviral drugs are commonly given prophylactically to prevent this.

The marrow shows signs of recovery usually within 2–3 weeks, and once the neutrophil count has begun to rise, restrictions, precautions, and supportive therapy can be relaxed. Without complications, transplant patients are in hospital for some 7–10 days pre-transplant and some 21–35 days afterwards.

11. Given no further problems, it takes some 2 months for the marrow and 6 months for the immune system to get back to normal. There is still a risk during this time of opportunist infections, and the immune deficiency experienced by marrow graft recipients, prolonged and worsened if graft-versus-host disease is troublesome, predisposes such children to the full spectrum of disease associated with lymphocyte functional deficiency (see Chapter 12).

# Compatibility for marrow transplantation—what does it mean?

Blood groups (i.e. red cell groups) and the transfusion of red cells have been briefly described in Chapter 12. Red cells are relatively simple compared with other cells in the body when it comes to transplanting them. There are only two cell characteristics (called antigens), that are usually of vital importance—the ABO group and the Rhesus type. There are just four ABO groups and two important basic Rhesus types.

White cells—including stem cells and cells of the immune system—are more complicated. They possess two major systems of antigens (roughly equivalent to red cell groups) called Class I and Class II. The problem is that there are over 50 different antigens making up Class I and over 20 in Class II, and each individual will have from two to four Class I antigens and two or more Class II. The potential number of combinations is therefore huge, though some antigens are much more common than others. The combination of these histocompatibility antigens, as they are called, is sometimes referred to as a tissue type or HLA type as the antigens involved are known as *human leucocyte antigens*. With such large numbers of possible types it can be readily appreciated that the chances of two people plucked at random from the street being compatible with each other from an HLA point of view is vanishingly small. (From a red cell point of view the figure would be roughly one in five or better.)

This is a pity because compatibility in terms of the HLA type is more important in bone marrow transplantation than other organ grafts. Mismatched kidneys and hearts can be tolerated if the host's immune response is muted by drugs, but following marrow transplants, the new immunity will never grow and function properly if it is locked in a state of civil war with the whole spectrum of organs in its own body. In the process of that war it may wreak irreparable damage on the organs most involved.

Fortunately it is not always necessary to rely on chance to find a suitable donor. The genes responsible for the histocompatibility antigens of any individual are in a tight cluster on chromosome number 6 called the *major histocompatibility complex* or MHC. Because they are close together, they are almost invariably inherited as a package, so two siblings have an approximately one in four chance of inheriting the same HLA type as each other. Patients from large families thus have an advantage when it comes to marrow transplantation. Parents, however, make less suitable donors, because they have only half of their histocompatibility antigens in common with any of their children, and half alike may not be alike enough for a successful marrow graft. The same goes for half brothers and sisters, and cousins, uncles, and aunts are similarly unlikely to be suitable.

For potential marrow recipients who have no matched brothers and sisters, it is useless recruiting a small number of volunteers and hoping one will prove, by chance, to have the same tissue type, despite the fact that some histocompatibility antigens are quite common. It is the *combination* of antigens that is important, and for adequate compatibility ideally most Class I and all Class II antigens have to match. The situation can be imagined as rather like a fruit machine with six large wheels and trying to get the same combination on two successive spins. The only way to find a compatible donor under such circumstances is to search large numbers of registered potential donors whose details are kept on computer databases by transfusion services or similar organizations. The likelihood of finding one depends on the rarity of the patient's HLA type and the size of the database consulted. For the commoner HLA types the chances will be good, but for rare types there is a less than one in 10 chance.

It is also possible to search the growing number of cord blood banks for suitable stem cells. The HLA type of cord blood does not have to be as good a match for Class I antigens as that of unrelated marrow donations. This is because the immature immune system of newborns is less likely to generate severe graft-versus-host disease than marrow from older children or adults with the same degree of HLA compatibility. Class II antigens still have to match.

If an unrelated donor or cord blood with the same broad HLA type is found, it is then usual to perform some further, more sophisticated, tests of compatibility comparing the Class II profile in minute detail. Some donors initially thought suitable may have to be rejected at this stage. Problems of graft failure and graft-versus-host disease tend to be greater with unrelated donors, so great care is needed. Results in children are improving, however, so it is now increasingly common practice to accept donors with a degree of mis-matching of Class I antigens where there is no alternative—including half-alike (or *haploidentical*) parents.

# Graft-versus-host disease

As already described, the commonest problem arising from incompatibility is not rejection of the transplant by the recipient, but attempted rejection of the recipient by the transplant—an attack on the host by the graft. This is because the transplant contains a new immune system as part of the package, and this new system, if not sufficiently similar to the one it is replacing, fails to recognize the body it is in as 'self'. The result is called *graft-versus-host disease* or GVH.

GVH can be trivial or fatal, and arise within a few days of the transplant or later. It can be a brief event with no after-effects, or a long-standing and disabling problem. Children are less troubled by it, on the whole, than adults, but occasionally it can provide major difficulties. It is best considered in two categories, acute and chronic.

## Acute GVH disease

This can occur up to 3 months after the transplant, but usually appears in the first 2–3 weeks. It causes a rise in temperature, rashes, jaundice, and diarrhoea. Fever and rashes are usual whereas the other features are more variable. The problem can be trivial, with a transient itching and redness of the skin (typically the palms and soles), or devastating with skin blistering, liver failure, and profuse diarrhoea.

It is treated either by high doses of steroids to suppress the inflammation or special serum to inactivate the responsible T lymphocytes. This may be followed by complete disappearance of the problem, improvement with persistent symptoms, or, rarely in the most severe cases, by no response and death. It is often difficult to be sure that acute GVH is just that and not an intercurrent virus or other infection (or both), and it is then helpful to take a small piece of affected skin for microscopic examination as the appearances of GVH can be recognized in this way.

Acute GVH is caused by mature T lymphocytes in the infused marrow that divide rapidly to launch an immediate attack. It can be avoided by removing the T lymphocytes from the marrow before infusion, and this is commonly done where acute GVH is most likely—when using unrelated donors. It is not *always* done, for two reasons. First, some leukaemias show a high relapse rate if transfused marrow is T lymphocyte depleted, and secondly, in most matched sibling transplants in children it is simply not necessary, as acute GVH is not commonly a serious problem.

## Chronic GVH disease

Chronic GVH is what the disease is called if it appears over 3 months after the transplant. It can follow straight on from the acute variety, may appear some time after an apparent complete resolution of it, or crop up on its own without any preceding symptoms and signs at all. It is perpetuated by a new generation of T cells that have grown from the transplant stem cells (rather than the pre-formed T cells in the transfused marrow), is much more indolent, and can go on for years.

It generates a type of permanent internal civil war perpetuated by the new immune system. It is so busy attacking its host it does not carry out its proper duties and offer protection from opportunistic infections. In other words chronic GVH disease produces a long-term immunodeficiency. It causes chronic skin disease with scarring and thickening, dry scabby eyes, and occasionally mild grumbling liver problems. It is difficult to treat, as long-term steroids are associated with unacceptable side-effects, but strangely *thalidomide*, better known for its terrible effects on developing babies, has a calming effect on the symptoms and signs of chronic GVH disease, and can be useful.

## Graft-versus-leukaemia effect

The idea that T cells help to prevent relapse ties up with the observation noted above that following an allogeneic marrow transplant for leukaemia there can be a beneficial effect additional to the simple 'rescue' role of the procedure. This has been called the 'graft-versus-leukaemia' effect. The theory behind it is that the new immune system eliminates any small remaining pockets of residual disease by a direct attack on the leukaemia cells. It is related to a GVH reaction, as evidenced by the fact that there is no suggestion of any graft-versus-leukaemia effect when identical twins are transplanted. (Such twins, of course, being totally compatible do not get GVH disease, but show a higher rate of relapse of the leukaemia despite transplantation.) The effect has been well summed up by the sentiment that 'a little GVH disease does you good'—with emphasis on the little.

# Autologous transplants—how they are done

The fundamental difference between an allogeneic transplant and an autologous procedure is that, in the latter, the patient's own (previously harvested and stored) marrow is used instead of that from another individual. It has the same advantage in that it allows the higher dosage schedules of chemotherapy and radiotherapy to be explored, and has the major attraction that there is no problem with finding a suitable donor. But, as far as leukaemia is concerned, the procedure has two major potential drawbacks. First, undetectable quantities of leukaemic cells could escape destruction by being in the marrow put on one side for re-infusion, and secondly, there can be no graft-versus-host reaction, so no added value of any graft-versus-leukaemia effect.

# The role of marrow transplantation in childhood leukaemia—who needs it?

Any marrow transplant, be it allogeneic, syngeneic, or autologous, carries a high price in terms of complications, some of which are fatal. So there is a large element of risk. Whether transplants can cure children with leukaemia depends, of course, on the type of leukaemia, the stage of the disease (first or subsequent remission), and the type of transplant (autologous, identical twin, matched sibling, cord blood, or unrelated donor). It also depends on the conditioning treatment.

The two questions that need to be clearly considered are these:

1. What are the chances of long-term survival and possible cure using conventional therapy without a transplant?

2. What are the chances of a transplant offering a real improvement in outlook?

If a child has newly encountered 'common' ALL without any adverse features, the answer to question 1 is excellent and to question 2 none. If the same child relapses on treatment, the answers change to poor and good respectively. If the same child has no transplant and two more relapses the answers change to nil and poor, and so on.

There is, of course, another uncontrollable variable in the equation, that being the availability of a suitable donor. There is no argument that, historically, the best results from any sort of transplant procedure have come from matched siblings. They usually provide sufficient compatibility to avoid major problems with GVH disease on the one hand, and just sufficient *in* compatibility to provide a graft-versus-leukaemia effect on the other.

Autologous transplants have not yet proved worthwhile in the control of either ALL or AML in childhood but may have a role in adult AML.

Unrelated donor transplants used to be rare events carried out only in centres with a major interest in their development. Now they have become more widely used, partly because the results have improved, partly because more donors are available on the international reg-istries, and partly because more centres now offer them as part of their portfolio of services. Cord blood transplants are also being carried out more often and it is likely that their popularity will grow.

So, presently, who should have what sort of transplant? Balancing risks and benefits but bearing in mind the lack of good evidence from randomized clinical trials, the following cautious generalizations might be made.

1. Matched sibling allogeneic transplants, if an option, should be considered for any child in remission from leukaemia whose prospect of 5-year disease-free survival with the best available conventional treatment is less than 50 per cent. This will include AMLs in first remission who do not have favourable features (see Chapter 11). It will include a small number of children with ALL in their first remission in the highest risk groups (see Chapter 8). It will include all children with relapsed leukaemia (if they have not had a transplant before), *except* perhaps those who initially had low risk ALL and who relapse over 12 months after completion of treatment.

2. Unrelated and/or mismatched donor transplants can now be considered for the same categories of patient, but many physicians are rather more cautious and would reserve their use for children in second or subsequent remissions only. The rules are changing quite rapidly, however, as results with unrelated matched and mis-matched donors are improving. It is difficult to generalize and every case has to be considered on its individual merits.

# Outcome of marrow transplantation

The main reason for failure of bone marrow transplantation for leukaemia is relapse of the basic disease despite everything. Added to that is the risk of death from the complications of the procedure (up to 10 per cent) which gives an overall disease-free long-term survival for the categories of patient described above of around 50 per cent. Long-term survivors also have a range of late effects of the process, which are described in Chapter 16. With greater experience these figures should improve.

## Donor lymphocyte infusions

If leukaemia relapses after bone marrow transplantation there is some-times the possibility of a second transplant, and repeating the whole exercise with a different donor. An alternative, however, is to attempt to provoke a graft-versus-leukaemia effect by deliberately inducing graft-versus-host disease from the original donor. The theory is that if the disease can be brought under control with conventional chemotherapy, a regenerated graft-versus-leukaemia reaction might suppress it sufficiently to produce long remissions.

The effect is achieved by collecting white cells from the original donor by apheresis (see Chapter 12) and then infusing some of these (in particular the mature T cells necessary to produce the graft-versus-host reaction) into the patient. The procedure is potentially hazardous, as there is a risk of producing a severe and life-threatening graft-versus-host reaction, but there have been some encouraging results in patients with adult-type chronic granulocytic leukaemia (see Chapter 14). So far the experience in children with more common types of leukaemia is limited and the technique is still regarded as highly experimental.

## Special centres for marrow transplantation

Like mis-matched allografts and donor lymphocyte infusions, many marrow transplant-based treatments are highly experimental and need corresponding experience and expertise not available in all children's cancer centres. For this reason children may have to travel to other hospitals where specialist units have been established. This will continue to be necessary until the value and role of some of the procedures involved have been established and they enter the realm of routine therapy.

# 14
# Uncommon leukaemias and diseases predisposing to leukaemia

## Uncommon leukaemias

All leukaemias in children are rare, but those that are not some type of ALL or AML are very unusual indeed. They comprise only around 2 per cent of the total. They are a miscellaneous group of disorders, falling into two broad categories. The first are easily recognizable as a form of leukaemia, whereas the second are characterized by disturbed bone marrow function causing lack of normal blood cell production without such an obvious accumulation of abnormal white cells. The first type includes the chronic leukaemias (more commonly seen in adults), and the second group is referred to collectively as the *myelodysplastic syndromes* (*myelo* = marrow, *dys* = disordered, *plastic* = growth).

## Chronic leukaemias

The terms *acute* and *chronic* simply refer to the natural time course of a disease and do not relate to how serious it is. Acute diseases last a short time, chronic diseases drag on. In terms of leukaemia the names refer to the progress of the disease in the untreated state, so acute leukaemias kill quickly, chronic varieties kill slowly. Except that now, because acute childhood leukaemias can be successfully treated, there is a paradoxical reversal, and the survival of children with some types of chronic leukaemia can be considerably shorter.

Chronic leukaemias differ in other respects than their speed of evolution. The white cells that are overproduced are more mature, and in many instances do not appear to be abnormal in appearance, just in numbers. They can be neutrophils and other granulocytes producing *chronic granulocytic* or *chronic myeloid leukaemia* (CGL, CML; same disease, different name), a mixture of granulocytes and monocytes (*chronic myelomonocytic leukaemia*, CMML) or lymphocytes (*chronic lymphocytic leukaemia*, CLL). Only CGL occurs as the same disease in both adults and children; CMML is very different in child-hood, and CLL in juveniles is so rare it could be said not to arise at all in the first two decades of life.

## Adult-type chronic granulocytic (myeloid) leukaemia

Adult-type CML (ATCML) in children is very infrequent. On average, in a city with a population of 500 000 a new case might arise every 10–12 years. It comes to light in a variety of ways, mostly insidi-ous, and is often discovered accidentally when children have a blood test for some other reason. It may declare itself through a growing pot belly caused by massive enlargement of the spleen, a hallmark of the disease. It can develop at any age. Typically there is a very high white blood cell count, but the cells look more or less normal, and there may not be any change in red cell numbers. Platelets can be low, normal, or high.

In its early stages ATCML can be difficult to distinguish from an abnormal response to infection—a leukaemia-like reaction, though the true disease does not go away, and the child is usually not so ill. Observation for a few weeks usually makes matters clear. If ATCML is left unchecked over several months, the white cell count can climb very high and then the blood gets sticky and fails to circulate pro-perly through the smallest blood vessels. This can cause drowsiness and impaired hearing, eventually leading to coma (*leucostasis*, also seen in AML and ALL, but with a more gradual onset in ATCML).

The diagnosis can be confirmed by the demonstration of a peculiar genetic corruption in the developing blood cells. This altered frag-ment of DNA is a reciprocal translocation of material from one chro-mosome (number 22) to another (number 9), and where the two fragments join on chromosome 22 a new (abnormal) gene is formed (called *BCR-ABL*) which produces a protein affecting cell growth. The corruption can be recognized if the chromosomes are studied under the microscope because the 22 chromosome looks small and stubby. In 1960 it was the first consistent chromosome abnormality to be recognized in human leukaemia and is named after the city of its discovery, Philadelphia. The Philadelphia chromosome does occur in a few acute leukaemias as well, but is present in some 95 per cent of cases of ATCML. Otherwise the marrow is just packed with normal-looking cells. Some cases are typical in every respect but lack the Philadelphia chromosome.

ATCML has two phases, benign and malignant. While the cells appear mature and bone marrow function is well preserved, excess white cell production can be controlled by oral drugs such as *busulphan* or *hydroxyurea*, or by regular injections of *interferon*. The oral drugs do not induce remission in the same way that drugs for acute leukaemia do, they merely suppress leukaemia cell production. Interferon is different in that a few patients will enter a true remission and the abnormal chromosome will disappear, sometimes for several years as long as the therapy is continued. Whether interferon can effect a cure is doubtful. In most patients in remission, although the Philadelphia chromosome may not be visible in the developing blood cells, using very sensitive laboratory techniques there is usually still evidence of low level activity of the *BCR-ABL* gene. This indicates that there are a few cells somewhere still carrying the abnormal chromosome and that the disease is dormant rather than eradicated.

On conventional therapy, benign-phase ATCML turns malignant (transforms) after a variable period of time—anything from 3 months to 10 years—with an average of 2–3 years. The result can look like AML or, surprisingly perhaps, like ALL, but is very difficult to treat successfully and subsequent survival is usually very short. Bone marrow transplantation early during the benign phase is presently the only therapy likely to allow long-term survival and cure in ATCML.

## Juvenile chronic myelomonocytic leukaemia (juvenile chronic myeloid leukaemia)

Chronic myelomonocytic leukaemia in children is so different from the nearest adult counterpart that it is prefixed by the word juvenile to distinguish it. The disorder is confined to childhood, has a predilection for males, and is commonest in toddlers. It occurs slightly less often than ATCML. It is often not recognized as a leukaemia in its early stages, though there is usually a high white cell count (with an excess of monocytes), a low platelet count, large lymph nodes, and a big spleen. Affected children get repeated infections and may bruise. Skin rashes are common. There are no distinguishing features in the bone marrow, and usually no chromosome abnormalities to help make the diagnosis.

A few patients have a benign variant that can fizzle out and allow long-term survival, but the classical syndrome is a very vicious disease with an average survival from diagnosis to death of less than a year. Affected children die of infection and bleeding from progressive marrow failure, but there is no clear two-phase component to JCMML as with ATCML. Bone marrow transplantation is the only treatment that has apparently cured occasional patients, though several have experienced recurrence after the transplant. Other therapies only temporarily alleviate the problem.

## Myelodysplastic syndromes

Myelodysplastic syndromes (MDS) is a useful but non-specific umbrella term that covers a variety of leukaemia-related disorders falling short of the full-blown disease. All are related, closely or more distantly, to AML. There are no recognized lymphodysplastic syndromes related to or preceding ALL. There are some diseases that predispose sufferers to develop leukaemia, both AML and ALL, but that is a different matter as the leukaemia then is an occasional complication rather than an advanced stage in the evolution of a disease. They will be considered separately.

Some MDS are well defined and their course and outlook known, others are more vague and it is not always clear how they are going to progress, if at all. Those that invariably precede obvious leukaemia used to be referred to as 'pre-leukaemia', and those that are recognizable as having some of the features of leukaemia but proceeding at a slow pace used to be called 'smouldering leukaemia'. These terms are no longer used but are illustrative of the tempo of MDS.

Myelodysplastic syndromes are much commoner in adults than children and particularly in the elderly. They have in common a degree of bone marrow failure and disturbance of normal blood cell production. Where the output of red cells, white cells, and platelets are *all* affected, the problem is referred to as *trilineage myelodysplasia*. They are grouped into three types with increasingly obvious features of leukaemia:

(a) refractory anaemia (RA);

(b) refractory anaemia with excess blasts (RAEB);

(c) refractory anaemia with excess blasts in transformation (RAEB-t).

There are two other types seen only in adults. One is refractory anaemia with ring sideroblasts (RARS), a variant of red cell dysplasia (RA) where the erythroblasts have iron granules in them. The other is *chronic myelomonocytic leukaemia* (CMML). It does not occur in children but has some similarities to JCMML (see above).

As the names suggest, the only fundamental difference between RA, RAEB, and RAEB-t is the degree to which the bone marrow is populated by potentially leukaemic blast cells. All are likely to produce marrow failure to the point where blood transfusions will be needed, but in RAEB-t the outlook is so poor that most physicians would proceed to treat them the same as full-blown AML without waiting for the disease to develop.

There is a specific recognizable childhood disorder where the marrow cells have lost one of the pair of chromosomes numbered 7, called *monosomy 7 syndrome*. Although this chromosome abnormality is not uncommon in leukaemic blast cells from patients of all ages with AML, in young infants, usually male, it is associated with a distinct syndrome that has some features in common with JCMML (see above). While the disease can run a time course of years, these unfortunate children develop marrow failure with enormous enlargement of the spleen or proceed to develop frank AML.

Monosomy 7 can arise without the features of CMML or greatly enlarged spleens, but if so is usually associated with myelodysplasia and usually progresses to frank AML.

# Diseases predisposing to leukaemia

There are several childhood diseases where there is an increased risk of the development of leukaemia. All are associated with a recognized defective gene or genes, either inherited or acquired at the time of conception. Most are rare, with two exceptions—Down syndrome and neurofibromatosis type 1 (von Recklinghausen's disease).

## Down syndrome

Down syndrome is associated with an extra copy of chromosome 21 in all cells in the body. The association between leukaemia and Down syndrome is 20 times more frequent than would be expected by chance. In addition to true leukaemia, Down children occasionally have a leukaemia-like picture around the time of birth (with high white cell counts and blast cells circulating in the blood) that can resolve spontaneously. It is described as a transient myelodysplasia and may never return. In infancy, however, there is also a peculiar predisposition to develop AML type M7 (see Chapter 10). Down children also develop ALL more frequently. This, and AML, respond quite satisfactorily to treatment, and it is now unusual for there to be any reluctance to offer leukaemia therapy to such children on the grounds of their basic handicap.

## Neurofibromatosis type 1 (von Recklinghausen's disease)

This inherited predisposition to develop multiple benign tumours (lumps) all over the body is quite common though is rarely expressed in such a spectacular form as the Elephant Man, perhaps the most famous sufferer. In its mildest form there may be no lumps, just one or more patches of skin discoloration like coffee stains. Sufferers are at a modestly increased risk of developing JCMML or AML. The reason is not known.

## Other diseases predisposing to leukaemia

There are several other very rare inherited disorders with a variable increased leukaemia risk, most of which are associated with disordered immunity or profoundly perturbed bone marrow function. Many are life threatening in their own right. In such patients the results of treating leukaemia are generally disappointing.

The disorders concerned include Fanconi's anaemia and Kostmann's severe congenital neutropenia (AML risk), Bloom's syndrome (ALL), ataxia telangiectasia (ALL and lymphomas), and Bruton-type agammaglobulinaemia (a lack of B cells and antibodies carrying an ALL/lymphoma risk). There are several other rare conditions where an increased leukaemia risk has been suspected but not substantiated.

# 15

# Coping with leukaemia

As well as the emotional trauma caused by a child with leukaemia there can be enormous practical problems for families. There is much travelling backwards and forwards to one or more hospitals, sometimes planned, sometimes not, and occasionally long and unanticipated periods away from home. This huge disruption to normal family life can generate psychological, financial, social, and employment difficulties for the parents, and the patient's brothers and sisters commonly get caught in the backwash.

Even when all seems to be going well, there is the ever-present fear of relapse, which is heightened at the successful completion of planned treatment, and then other worries creep in about long-term effects of treatment, fertility, and future generations (see Chapter 16). For the unlucky children who do relapse there is the anxiety and despair this produces coupled with more treatment, more travelling, and more time in hospital often accompanied by a dwindling hope of success. Finally there may eventually be the prospect of bereavement, preceded by the anguish where all hope of cure has gone. Practical difficulties can be an added burden at such times.

Each patient is unique in terms of the type and stage of their disease. Each family is also unique in their geographic, social and financial circumstances, ethnic background, and personalities. For this reason it is very difficult to generalize about the problems they will face, and to unpick the intricate relationship between emotional and practical problems. But there are some aspects of living with leukaemia, both for the afflicted families and for the staff who care for them, about which it may be helpful to make some broad observations.

## Coping with treatment

### Emotional coping

Emotional problems are almost inevitable when people are faced with a severe threat over a long term. I call it the Damocles syndrome.

Damocles served at the court of Dionysius of Syracuse and openly envied his King's position so much that the King invited him to change places. A banquet was arranged at which Damocles was placed in the King's seat. Above him a razor-sharp sword was suspended by a single horse's hair, symbolizing the King's insecurity. Damocles was terrified to stir. The Sword of Damocles has thus come to represent a persistent and paralysing threat. For parents of children with leukaemia, the sword is suspended at diagnosis. It should gradually disappear as time slips by following successful completion of treatment, though for some it still inappropriately hangs there, many years later.

## Coping with the diagnosis

The initial shock of learning the diagnosis is similar for all parents, irrespective of the type of leukaemia. Most will have heard of it, will be aware that it is a cancer of the blood, and that it is potentially fatal. Breaking the news is best done in stages. First, the fact must be accepted. Secondly, and preferably some time later after the initial shock has subsided, the full diagnosis and outlook should be explained.

Initial questions often reflect irrational guilt about being in some way responsible for the disease by error or omission, and sometimes parents try to relate the problem to some event, usually an injury. Several informal question and answer sessions will be needed in the early days, and then gradually families will settle into focusing on the practical problems of treatment delivery and complications.

A hurdle sometimes encountered at the time of diagnosis is gaining informed consent for entry into clinical trials that require an early randomization to different treatments. The nature and structure of such trials is considered in Chapter 7. It is difficult enough for parents to come to terms with the fact of leukaemia. It is unrealistic to expect them easily and quickly to understand fully the complexities of clinical trials and the need for them. The attitude 'I'm not interested in experiments, I want the best treatment whatever that is' is quite reasonable under the circumstances. What needs to be explained, therefore, is that *every* treatment schedule for leukaemia is experimental and whether a protocol or plan is part of a formal clinical trial or not does not alter this fact. This will be true until 100 per cent of children can be cured without fuss or any side effects.

It is also helpful to understand that the remarkable progress in the last 20 years has been mostly as a result of experimental treatments studied in the context of clinical trials, and that in the past children in such trials have generally fared better than those excluded, for whatever reason. Parents also need to understand that they are benefiting from children in previous trials and that the debt can be settled by their own child's contribution to the welfare of those that will follow. They need to appreciate that trial questions focus on real areas of uncertainty and that if one treatment appears to be better than another as the trial proceeds, then all children will be immediately switched to the best option. Despite the difficulties, most parents agree to enter trials, and in the ensuing days as their level of understanding grows, the number that regret their decision is negligible.

Emotional problems experienced by the children themselves will depend, of course, on their age. Infants are concerned about being separated from their parents, and children up to the age of 8 or 10 are more worried about the day-to-day physical discomfort of treatment than the broader issues of cure or death. It is only older children and adolescents who really care about what is wrong with them rather than what is being done to them. The majority prefer their options in black and white rather than shades of grey. Most respond best to being told that they have leukaemia, that if they do not have treatment they will not get better and (if they ask the question) they may die, but that if they do go through the treatment they will eventually be cured. It is never helpful to trivialize the problem and imply that the disease is not serious, because that will not tie up with the unpleasant and extended treatment, and creates a barrier of distrust between patient and attendants.

## Settling down during treatment

As treatment proceeds, the amazing adaptability of human beings shows through and life usually settles into an uneasy routine. Many parents will become thoroughly familiar with the disease pattern and treatment schedules and will eventually, for example, question prescriptions, suggest the need for transfusions, and scrutinize blood counts. They will become friendly with other parents, nurses, and doctors, often on first name terms. By doing so they will become part of a new social order, an exclusive cabal from which mutual support can be gained. As Bacon said, adversity is not without comforts and hopes. But some parents will remain private and detached.

The informal parental camaraderie is a spawning ground for organized groups common to many children's cancer centres. These parent-driven initiatives usually become registered charities, raise funds for patient support and research, and sometimes become quite large, handling large amounts of money and employing nurses, social workers, and doctors. They commonly have large numbers of members, only a few of who are active in running their committees. There is much genuine altruism, but it is also fair to say that many of those heavily involved derive much personal satisfaction. Some bereaved parents find solace in this way.

As treatment progresses the problems encountered by ALL sufferers diverge somewhat from those met by patients with AML. In ALL, the long drawn-out phase of maintenance therapy over 2 years with regular visits to the clinic and daily tablet taking can, if uneventful, become tedious. Adolescents particularly can resent being different from their peers, and may deny their disease, feeling well as they do. They may fail to take all their medication. Much less commonly, parents may also tire of the routine of tablet taking and relax their efficiency.

AML patients face different problems. The pattern for them is a shorter time-scale of repeated hospital admissions for unpleasant pulses of chemotherapy, commonly followed by further time in hospital receiving supportive measures for therapy-induced bone marrow failure. They have only occasional brief interludes of healthy remission at home before the cycle repeats itself—usually four to five times, with or without a bone marrow transplant. Again, it is the adolescents who have the biggest problem coping with the intense disruption to their lives and the unpleasant bouts of deliberately induced illness.

## Other problems during treatment

Some families have much worse emotional difficulties during therapy than most other families. These are often precipitated by unexpected major complications when children become extremely ill and nearly die, or by a continuing stormy clinical course with repeated hospital admissions for intercurrent problems when most patients are home and well. Mothers who are socially isolated at home also sometimes suffer extra distress. Marriage difficulties are not unusual, and parental alcohol abuse is also common.

Important behaviour problems can arise in the patients themselves and/or their siblings. It is easy to say that children with leukaemia should be treated normally, but very hard to apply in practice. Not surprisingly, feeding off the adult anxiety and attention around them, some young sufferers become skilled emotional manipulators and end up with their parents (and grandparents) tied in knots and pandering to their every whim. In such circumstances the stage is set for ignored siblings to go off the rails.

## Completion of treatment

The successful completion of treatment is a difficult time for parents, as they lose the 'crutch' of medication, and enter a fingers-crossed, wait-and-see phase. Most children who are going to relapse will do so during the first 18 months of therapy, and watching and waiting is an understandably stressful time.

## Practical coping

Treatment schedules for leukaemia are all complicated, and progress through them is punctuated by stop–go periods dictated by low blood counts or intercurrent problems. There will be many trips to hospital and for some families without their own transport this can be very disruptive and expensive. Most employers are very sympathetic and flexible in allowing their staff time off, though it can be difficult for small organizations, or self-employed parents, and sometimes loss of income cannot be avoided.

## Social worker support

All children's cancer centres should have the services of specialist social workers whose job it is (amongst other things) to help with practical advice and help (including financial help) when families experience difficulties. Such staff are familiar with leukaemia and its treatment, and have much technical knowledge. They are also familiar with the charitable organizations that can provide help, and with the assistance available from various government sources. They work very closely with specialist nurses and doctors.

## Shared care

The need for shared care between hospitals has been discussed in Chapter 12. Where this works well it is excellent. There is always, however, a risk of running back to the main centre when things go wrong, or are perceived to go wrong. It is important to generate trust in parents and children and for all staff at the main centre to instil confidence that shared care centres are completely competent.

## School

There is no good medical reason why children with leukaemia in remission who are well enough to be at home should not go to school in the normal way. The risk of infection they run is not much increased by mixing with their peers, and the benefits of going to school are considerable. Despite this there is a tendency on the part of parents to be over-protective. There is also a nervousness on the part of teachers, and these factors combine to keep patients off school for no good reason, or (for example) to allow strapping teenagers to go for only half days so that they do not get 'too tired'.

Part of the problem is due to exaggeration of the risks of chicken-pox (see Chapter 12), a disease that is endemic in schools. It cannot be over-emphasized that the occasions when it is justified to keep a child with leukaemia (in remission on treatment) away from school on the grounds of other pupils' illnesses are very few and far between.

Children themselves may not want to go back to school after their first absence, particularly if they have started to lose their hair—a temporary side-effect of the chemotherapy and radiotherapy. This understandable self-consciousness and reluctance should be gently and sympathetically overcome. The great majority of patients can be successfully renaturalized into school society without difficulty given a little determination.

There are, of course, odd exceptions to the 'fit for home, fit for school' rule which can be defined by common sense. *Short* periods of convalescence after major periods of illness, or a bone marrow transplant, are perhaps permissible. And terminal care, seldom a long process in children with leukaemia, may demand peace and quiet, though having school friends and teachers to visit even at that stage is never a bad thing.

## Social interplay

Occasionally families wrestling with leukaemia can find themselves increasingly isolated, and the affected children can lose their normal social contacts in informal day-to-day play as well as at schooltime. The problem is the product of many factors; protectiveness by the sufferer's parents worried about infection, awkwardness on the part of friends or friends' parents not knowing how to approach the affected child, and (rarely) fear of contagion. Every effort should be made to avoid it happening. Children deprived of peer contact of this type are much more at risk of psychological disturbance.

# Coping with treatment failure

Relapse at any time is devastating news. Given current salvage treatment, some children who relapse late, after the first programme of treatment has finished, will still become long survivors, but probably no more than 50 per cent. For those who relapse early, on treatment or within 6 months of its completion, the outlook is much more gloomy (see Chapters 9 and 11). Most of those who relapse for a second or third time, or after a bone marrow transplant, have little chance of long-term disease-free survival whatever treatment is given. For them there may be no realistic hope of cure and this has to be faced.

At what stage the parents and patients (and their attendants) accept the unacceptable depends on individual circumstances. Facing the incurability of a particular child does not necessarily or usually imply impending death. Palliative treatment may maintain remission for months or occasionally years. And at any time the option to try some novel therapy can be revisited. For the children themselves, the decision to palliate is a stage that can be rationalized as one where the disease is incurable but can be controlled by continuing medication—like diabetes. Most can be reconciled to that concept.

As parents struggle to come to terms with their coming loss, they may go through several stages. 'Somebody somewhere must be able to do something' is a common reaction. The options for further treatment should be explored in a rational and calm way, and the pros and cons of pursuing one or other thoroughly mulled over. There may be an opportunity to enter trials of new drugs under development where the activity against leukaemia is being assessed in phase 1 and phase 2 clinical drug trials (see Chapter 7). If so, it should be appreciated that there is no realistic prospect of cure using these experimental compounds, rather there is a chance of some disease control, possible partial remission, and a short extension of life expectancy with good quality of life. By the nature of these studies, there is, of course, no guarantee of a good result, and there may be unexpected side effects. The pros and cons should be weighed up carefully in each individual case.

Towards the end the needs of the patient and the parents may diverge. When all reasonable hope of achieving any benefit from aggressive treatment has gone, the child's interests dictate that he/she should be treated in a minimalist way to preserve health and keep him/her out of hospital as much as possible. The aim should be for the highest possible quality of life for whatever time is left. Some parents may have difficulty with that approach, and thrash around wanting more and more treatment, to 'leave no stone unturned' or 'go down with all guns blazing'. Others may seek solace in alternative medicine or faith-healing. Much of this is at least harmless and comfortable for the child, but sadly there are opportunists around willing to exploit parental distress and charge large amounts of money.

At such a time it is often helpful for parents to go to another cancer centre to talk to a disinterested specialist in an attempt to gain a better perspective of their plight. It can help them brace themselves for what is to come.

# Coping with death

How children with leukaemia go through the process of dying is, of course, very variable. Some of the physical aspects are described in Chapter 7. Compared with other childhood cancers, one of the few good things about leukaemia is that there is seldom a long drawn-out terminal bedridden phase. Also it is not, generally, a physically painful disease where massive doses of pain-killing drugs are needed, though generalized bone pain does arise in some children and modest doses of morphine or similar can help to keep them active in the last few weeks. With a little luck and skill, it is often possible to keep children dying from leukaemia reasonably well and enjoying life until a day or two before the end.

Parents preparing themselves for the death have understandable fears about how they will cope, what exactly will happen, and when. The children themselves seldom ask at this stage if they are going to die. For older children who have a perception of death, they may know but usually choose not to discuss it. Humans have an infinite capacity for self-deception, and it is very unusual for children to be obsessed by the possibility of their impending death.

Sometimes the death occurs at home, sometimes in hospital. This may be at the parents' wish, or dictated by the circumstances of the final event. If there have been any unexpected circumstances, or if there are puzzling features about the disease, it may be appropriate to consider a post-mortem examination, or *autopsy*. This will provide more information about the individual child, which the parents may find helpful in the future when trying to understand the past. It may also advance medical knowledge.

At the time of death it is common for grieving parents to say no to a request for a post-mortem, on the grounds that their child has 'suffered enough'. They may be resolute in their refusal, which is always respected. Sometimes they can be persuaded to agree to a limited examination of a particular organ of interest—the lungs, perhaps. Occasionally, where a post-mortem is likely to be especially important, the matter can be gently raised before death so that the parents are prepared and have time to think about it. Parents who agree to the procedure rarely regret it. They invariably derive benefit from eventually learning more about their child's death, and this helps them to come to terms with their loss.

# How staff cope

Parents and families are not, of course, the only ones affected by their child's leukaemia. There are many members of the hospital staff who will become closely involved, including nurses, doctors, social workers, nursery nurses, laboratory workers, X-ray workers, secretaries, porters, and domestic staff. Some will be young and relatively inexperienced, others more used to the strains dealing with potentially fatal diseases can bring. The job is not an easy one.

Many cancer centres run informal staff support groups to help with problems. There is a well-recognized problem of 'burn-out' in staff involved with childhood leukaemia for many years that needs to be recognized and dealt with when it occurs. It is characterized by increasing difficulty in the delivery of bad news and a degree of detachment. Such staff should move back from the front line and occupy a more administrative role, though this tends to happen with increasing seniority anyway. The time taken for the problem to develop (it happens in all long-serving medical and nursing staff to some extent) is variable, but 15 years directly in the bedside firing line should probably not be exceeded.

# 16

# The after-effects of leukaemia and its treatment

Nowadays most children with leukaemia survive their ordeal and grow to adulthood. That may not be the end of the story for them, however. There are still some problems that can arise, both physical and psychological. And for the unlucky ones who succumb to their disease, the parents and other family members will face the difficulties of bereavement. Either way, leukaemia can leave a legacy.

## Problems for survivors

### The late effects of treatment

Chemotherapy and radiotherapy are poisonous and destructive, and applying such drastic measures to growing children might be expected to cause untold damage to normal health and development. So it is perhaps surprising that for the great majority of patients the long-term effects of treatment for leukaemia are not clinically important and, indeed, for most there are none of note. It is essential to get the potential problems and risks into perspective to avoid unnecessary anxiety.

Another important point is that late effects being seen early in the twenty-first century relate to treatment schedules given in the 1970s to the 1990s. Some of the routine practices in earlier studies, particularly the more widespread application of radiation therapy, are no longer relevant, so the pattern of late effects may be changing.

### A second cancer

The worst thing that can happen to a long survivor of childhood leukaemia is to develop a second cancer—either another (different) leukaemia or a tumour of some other type.

The possibility of a second leukaemia arises because some of the drugs used in treating the first one can cause damage to the marrow stem cells leading to genetic corruption and the formation of abnormal chromosomes and genes (as described in Chapter 2). The drugs that can do this are cyclophosphamide, anthracyclines, and podophyllins (see Chapters 7 and 11). These secondary leukaemias are described in Chapter 10. They are very difficult to treat, but fortunately are very rare. Limiting the use of drugs known to cause the problem has further diminished the risk.

As far as other cancers are concerned, there is a statistically increased risk of ALL survivors developing brain tumours, particularly in those who have had radiation therapy to the head under the age of 5 years. This amounts to a 20-fold excess of the normal incidence. Whether the risk is entirely related to radiation is not clear. Cranial radiation has also very rarely been implicated in the development of thyroid cancer. Isolated examples of other tumours have been described but whether they represent a late effect of leukaemia treatment or just coincidence is far from certain.

Overall, the cumulative risk of some second malignant disease in long survivors of childhood leukaemia is hard to calculate accurately, but is probably of the order of 2–3 per cent at 20 years after finishing treatment. Remember, though, that this is likely to be an overestimate as it is based on observation of patients treated with more exposure to radiation and other therapies likely to cause cancer than those undergoing treatment at the present time.

Happily, there is presently nothing to suggest that offspring of long survivors are at any increased risk of leukaemia or other cancers.

## Late heart failure

Anthracycline drugs, although very effective against leukaemia, can damage the heart muscle and impair its function. This may not be apparent at the time and may not be discovered until some years later when the heart can suddenly fail. Heart failure simply means that its function as a pump falters and the amount of blood coming back to it is not matched by the amount it is able to pump out again. This is potentially serious and causes congestion of the lungs and liver. The damage is irreversible and means that in the worst cases a heart transplant has to be considered.

Since the problem has been recognized, however, it has virtually disappeared. This is because great care is taken to keep the amount of anthracycline drugs used as small as possible, to check on heart function very carefully, and to use special formulations or other drugs to protect the heart from the damaging effect of the drug. Despite all these precautions, occasional cases still arise, particularly in children with AML who have relapsed and been successfully salvaged with a second programme of therapy incorporating a bone marrow transplant.

## Growth and hormonal disorders

Long survivors of ALL are prone to short stature, obesity, and (in girls) premature puberty. This is because of disturbed function of the pituitary gland, a tiny organ at the base of the brain that has the important function of producing a variety of hormones (blood-carried chemicals) directly or indirectly controlling growth, metabolism (the body's energy consumption), and the function of the sex organs.

The pituitary is intimately linked to the brain and very vulnerable to damage from radiation treatment and (to a lesser extent) drugs used for treatment of the central nervous system (CNS). This can result in a lack of growth hormone, which reduces the height to which a child grows. It also influences the deposition of body fat, resulting in a tendency to chubbiness. Pituitary damage can cause premature signals to the immature ovary to start producing female sex hormones and eggs, resulting in premature or precocious puberty. Early puberty causes the growing bone ends to fuse and stop growing, compounding the effect on final height.

Damage to the pituitary is of variable severity and the effects are not an all-or-none affair. Minimal changes are not uncommon, but major problems of growth deficiency are rarely seen. This is more so since the move away from higher doses of radiation therapy to the brain, and the growth problems of children who receive no radiation are generally trivial.

The spinal growth problems seen in children treated in the 1970s with radiation treatment to the spine as well as the head now rarely occur as this practice has been largely discontinued. Some children's cancer groups still use it for children with leukaemia in the CNS. The effect on growth is due to direct damage of the growing bones of the spinal column. Affected children show disproportion with long arms and legs and a short trunk.

## Fertility

Women treated as children for ALL with current standard protocols are generally capable of conceiving and carrying uneventful pregnancies to term without difficulty. The same probably applies to AML survivors. Those who have had bone marrow transplants, however, will be infertile if total body radiation has been used as conditioning treatment (see bone marrow transplants, below).

Male fertility may be impaired by any leukaemia treatment at any age, and is rather hard to predict in any given case. Some long survivors have successfully fathered children, but the testis seems more vulnerable to chemotherapy than the ovary. The production of testosterone (the male sex hormone) is not usually disturbed, so boys go through puberty normally and are not impotent. Boys who have testicular radiation therapy, however, will be infertile and will need testosterone supplements. There was a period in the 1970s when this was standard practice, but now it is only applied if the testicles become directly involved with leukaemia (see Chapter 9). The dose of radiation used for bone marrow transplantation will cause sterility and may cause testosterone deficiency.

## Intellect and learning

Children surviving leukaemia may have difficulties at school and in their academic development. This is a complex problem, and not just due to late side-effects, though undoubtedly CNS-directed treatment can play a major part. The matter is currently being intensively researched to discover the respective roles of different components of treatment, but top of the list of potential villains is undoubtedly radiation therapy to the brain.

It was apparent many years ago that radiation therapy to the brains of children under the age of 2 was responsible for substantial intellectual dulling to the point of mental handicap. Older children, however, seemed not to suffer to anything like the same extent, and since the treatment was so evidently effective at preventing CNS relapse, the risks were considered to be outweighed by the benefits. Now alternative strategies are being employed, though whether high-dose methotrexate (for example) is less risky in terms of intellectual damage is not yet clear.

The greatest brain damage occurs in children who have a combination of relapsed CNS leukaemia, radiation treatment (sometimes two separate courses), and a large cumulative dose of methotrexate into the spinal fluid by lumbar puncture. All three components seem to play a part. Few such children become long survivors, but they tell us that the problem is multifactorial. All that can be said is that long survivors, as a group, may have an intellectual performance that is slightly but measurably less than their peers, but fortunately this is not a big problem for most individuals. Many successfully complete tertiary education and achieve high academic levels.

## Late effects of bone marrow transplantation

The catalogue of late effects after otherwise successful bone marrow transplantation is rather more daunting. Apart from chronic graft-versus-host disease, the problems are similar in type to those of children surviving conventional treatment but differ mostly in degree. They depend on the type of conditioning treatment, and total body radiation is a major factor in this respect.

Pre-pubertal whole body radiation recipients mostly show growth failure and some need growth hormone treatment. At any age whole body radiation can cause cataracts (due to damage to the lens of the eye causing it to go cloudy and hindering vision), and patients can develop under-functioning of the thyroid gland. All will be sterile and boys may need testosterone supplements at puberty and for life afterwards. Many will show intellectual dulling, though only to a disabling degree in a few.

Chronic graft-versus-host disease is a miserable problem and can severely impair the quality of life for survivors. It is a permanent state of civil war between the donor immune system and the recipient's skin, liver, lungs, and other organs. It causes a paradoxical immune deficiency state and exposes sufferers to the risk of overwhelming infections. If severe, it can itself shorten life expectancy.

## Psychological problems for long survivors

It is all too easy to concentrate on the fact that the leukaemia survivor is lucky to be alive and to have escaped with few late effects of treatment to worry about. In so doing you forget that there is a lot of mental adjustment for such patients to make as they face the rest of their lives and as they negotiate the turbulence of adolescence and young adulthood. Such times are difficult for normal children, but for those with real or perceived physical handicaps they are doubly so. It is not uncommon for leukaemia survivors, particularly girls, to feel 'different' and to feel very self-conscious with a distorted body image and low self-esteem.

Fears about fertility and sexual adequacy can compound the problem. All these worries may not become apparent at routine clinic visits where time is short, but a little patience can sometimes uncover a cauldron of psychological difficulties which need careful and sympathetic attention to help to alleviate.

Parents, too, can fail to make the adjustment back to normal and may fall prey to an extended Damocles syndrome (see Chapter 15). This can manifest itself as over-protectiveness and a reluctance to let children explore their own horizons long after treatment has finished.

# Problems of bereavement

The way parents and families cope with the loss of a child is unique to them, influenced by the type of people they are, their ethnic, religious and social background, the age of the child, and the circumstances of the loss. Many books have been written on the topic, and there is no place in this one for an extensive consideration of the matter, but there are a few points worth mentioning.

## Early unexpected deaths

If a child dies in the first few days following the diagnosis of leukaemia, the parents have special difficulties because they are still struggling to come to terms with the fact and nature of the disease as well as being unprepared for their child's death. For them, especially, it is important that they return after a few weeks to go over the sequence of events, to have the disease explained again, and to be reassured that what happened was unavoidable. The 'if onlys' need to be discussed. The anger commonly felt, sometimes undirected, sometimes focused on those perceived to be responsible for any delay in diagnosis, needs to be dissipated.

## Late unexpected deaths

Children who die in remission from some unanticipated inter-current infection can similarly leave parents unprepared, and the findings of a post-mortem examination can be especially useful in helping to answer some of the questions that inevitably arise.

## Expected deaths

Parents who have had some time to prepare themselves can still feel great bewilderment and confusion when the event occurs. They often repeatedly replay in their minds the last few days or hours, like a slow motion film, concentrating on every detail and puzzling whether (for example) a particular injection given at a particular time had materially altered the course of events. They require much reassurance that they did not fail their child in any way.

## Loss of social contact

Parents who have been attending a children's cancer centre for some years can suddenly find that their child's death precipitates the loss of regular companionship provided by hospital staff, other parents, and children, who have become a surrogate extended family for them. This can aggravate their struggle to pick up the pieces, and they feel a need to maintain some sort of contact. This might be by a frenzy of energetic fund-raising or offering 'support' to other parents through involvement with hospital-based parent groups.

## Bereavement counselling

Children's cancer centres seldom have the resources to provide a full counselling service for bereaved parents, but many support or encourage groups to meet for informal mutual psychotherapy. Most will suggest that those who have lost children return after a few months for at least one formal interview with the consultant physician in charge to discuss again the course of the illness and, as far as possible, to answer the inevitable question 'why?'

# For the future

Until every child with leukaemia can be cured without any late side-effects, there will be a continuing need for research and clinical trials. This activity will become more and more expensive and the returns for effort will diminish as the goal of 100 per cent problem-free survival is approached. The state-funded treatment of childhood leukaemia is beyond the resources of all but the wealthiest nations, and even there the cost is hard to meet when other diseases compete for limited government funds.

But this must be placed into a global context. World-wide, many more children die of leukaemia due to lack of access to adequate treatment than through relapsed or resistant disease. For them, current therapy programmes would allow a huge improvement in outlook if only there were some way to make them available. They provide the greatest challenge.

# A glossary of terms

**acute**: a disease running a rapid course.

**agglutination**: the process when blood cells stick together after (for example) transfusing blood of the wrong group.

**ALL**: acute lymphoblastic leukaemia.

**allogeneic transplant (allograft)**: a transplant of an organ from one genetically different individual to another.

**AML**: acute myeloid leukaemia.

**anaemia**: low blood haemoglobin concentration.

**ANLL**: acute non-lymphoblastic leukaemia.

**antibiotics**: drugs used to kill invading micro-organisms.

**antibody**: the parts in blood responsible for recognizing invaders.

**antigen**: the 'label' on a cell which is recognized by *antibodies*.

**apoptosis**: the orderly death of a cell as it shuts down its chemical activities under the control of in-built suicide genes.

**aspiration cytology**: microscopic examination of cells removed from (for example) bone marrow by suction through a hollow needle.

**autologous transplant (autograft)**: a procedure where bone marrow from an individual is stored outside the body for later replacement.

**benign**: not harmful.

**biopsy**: removal of a small amount of tissue for microscopic examination.

**blast cell**: an immature cell at an early stage of development.

**blood count**: numerical measurement of blood cells and haemoglobin concentration.

**blood groups**: genetically determined differences between red blood cells from different individuals.

**blood transfusion**: giving of blood, or some part of the blood, from one individual to another.

**bone marrow**: the organ system responsible for the production of blood cells.

**bone marrow transplantation**: as blood transfusion but using bone marrow rather than blood.

**CD; cluster of differentiation**: a feature of white blood cells indicating what type they are.

**CGL:** chronic granulocytic leukaemia (same as CML).

**chemotherapy:** drugs that are toxic to cancer cells.

**chromosomes:** short compact pieces of DNA that replicate and divide as cells multiply. Normal cells have 23 pairs.

**chronic:** a disease running a long slow course.

**clone:** a group of cells derived from, and similar to, a single cell of origin.

**CML:** chronic myeloid leukaemia (same as CGL).

**CNS:** central nervous system—the brain and spinal cord.

**coagulation:** the process of blood clotting and forming a solid jelly.

**commensal bacteria:** microbes that live in or on the body and normally cause no disease.

**compatibility:** similarity in genetic make-up between individuals necessary for successful blood transfusion or bone marrow transplantation.

**cross-match test:** a laboratory assessment of the suitability of red blood cells for transfusion into a given individual.

**cytopenia:** lack of cells (type unspecified).

**cytotoxic drugs:** cell-killing medication.

**DNA:** deoxyribonucleic acid—the part of every body cell (capable of replication) that contains the entire genetic code of the individual. Contained in 23 pairs of chromosomes.

**endemic:** always around in a particular geographical region, though perhaps not very common.

**enzymes:** body chemicals that facilitate essential chemical reactions.

**epidemic:** a sudden and large outbreak of a particular disease in a particular geographical region.

**erythrocyte:** red blood cell—contains haemoglobin, which carries oxygen all around the body.

**fever:** a rise in body temperature to above-normal levels.

**gene:** a tiny fragment of DNA that codes for a particular body chemical.

**genetic mutation:** corruption of a gene or genes during the process of cell reproduction.

**granulocyte:** a major subtype of white blood cell that includes neutrophils.

**haemoglobin:** a bright red compound in red blood cells that carries oxygen around the body.

**homologous transplant (homograft):** *see* allogeneic transplant.

**hyperdiploid:** cells containing more than the normal 46 chromosomes.

**immunophenotype**: characteristics of white blood cells recognized by specially made anti-cell antibodies.

**immune system**: the body's natural defences against micro-organisms or foreign tissue.

**inflammation**: a localized reaction to infection or invasion manifest by heat, pain, redness, and swelling. Sometimes accompanied by a rise in body temperature.

**JCMML; JCML**: juvenile chronic myelomonocytic leukaemia; juvenile chronic myeloid leukaemia.

**leucocyte**: the collective name for all types of white blood cells.

**leucostasis**: blockage of blood flow due to sludging caused by a huge excess of white blood cells.

**lumbar puncture**: insertion of a needle into the fluid around the base of the spinal cord at the bottom of the backbone.

**lymphatic system**: an organ system concerned with refuse disposal and immunity.

**lymph node**: a bean-sized collection of lymphocytes; part of the lymphatic system.

**lymphoblast**: a lymphocyte still at the developing stage.

**lymphocyte**: a type of white blood cell that is responsible for the body's immune system.

**lymphoma**: a cancer involving lymphocytes and the lymphatic system but not the bone marrow.

**macrophage**: general name for a blood cell which scavenges foreign material.

**malignant**: cancerous—growing into and damaging the surrounding tissues.

**micro-organism; microbe**: generic terms for bacteria, viruses, or fungi.

**mitosis**: the process of cell division into two identical cells.

**monocyte**: a type of white blood cell that develops into a *macrophage*.

**monosomy**: one of a pair of chromosomes is missing in a cell.

**myeloid**: literally 'marrow-like'; usually applied to cells indicating them to be of or from the marrow, or to leukaemia to indicate that it is not lymphocyte related.

**necrosis**: disorderly cell death by lack of blood supply or physical damage resulting in content spillage.

**neutropenia**: lack of neutrophils, predisposing to infection.

**neutrophil**: a type of white blood cell that ingests and destroys bacteria and other foreign material.

**oncogene**: a gene caused by DNA mutation that promotes or allows disorderly cell growth.

**oncology**: the science of the study of cancer.

**opportunistic infection**: an infection due to a germ that can only really take hold when the immune system is already weakened for some other reason.

**pancytopenia**: lack of all types of blood cell simultaneously.

**parenteral nutrition**: intravenous feeding.

**phagocytosis**: the action of a cell such as a neutrophil when it engulfs and destroys (for example) an invading microbe.

**plasma**: the straw-coloured fluid in which blood cells are suspended, and in which antibodies and other important chemicals are dissolved.

**platelets**: tiny cells that promote blood clotting by sticking to each other.

**prognosis**: the likely outcome of an illness.

**radiotherapy**: using a type of X-ray to kill cancer cells.

**red cells**: blood cells containing haemoglobin.

**relapse**: recurrence of a disease that had previously been inactive.

**remission**: the time when a disease is inactive but when there is the possibility of a relapse.

**risk factors**: features of a disease indicative of its likely response (or lack of it) to treatment.

**sanctuary site**: part of the body with an anatomical barrier to noxious chemicals in the bloodstream such as cytotoxic drugs.

**septicaemia**: bacteria growing in the bloodstream; sometimes called blood poisoning.

**serum**: clear cell-free fluid expressable from clotted blood.

**syngeneic transplant**: transplantation of organs between identical twins.

**trephine biopsy**: a small core of bone marrow removed with a circular cutting tool for microscopic analysis.

**white cells**: colourless blood cells of various types (*see* granulocyte, lymphocyte, monocyte, and neutrophil).

# Index

Page numbers in *italics* refer to figures.